Keto Diet Cookbook For Women Over 50:

Complete Guide for Senior Women. Lose up to 15lbs in 3 Weeks With 100+ Quick & Simple Keto Recipes & Easy to Follow 28-Day Meal Plan

AUTHOR
CLAIRE MILLER

Table of Contents

Introduction

Among the stars of the world show business and ordinary women, the keto diet is trendy. Few people know that initially, in the 20th century, it was used to treat epileptic seizures in children. A little later, doctors managed to establish that it is possible to significantly reduce the amount of fat by adhering to a keto diet. Now, this method of losing weight is one of the most effective and safe for health.

Keto-diet has other names: ketogenic, ketotic. Its essence is to achieve a state of ketosis, that is, the process of producing ketone bodies that carry energy with a lack of glucose in the blood. A food style is formed in simple words in which sugar is lowered, which forces the body to receive energy from fat stores.

Eating chocolate enhances mental and physical abilities. But the simple carbohydrates it contains increase glucose levels, which can cause diabetes and contribute to the deposition of fats on different parts of the body. If they do not come with food, the body will begin to draw energy from its reserves, actively absorbing fats.

Ketones are mainly produced by the liver from fat stores and are vital for the body. A similar condition is observed with a complete rejection of food. But if starvation is dangerous to health and life, a keto diet, on the contrary, is useful for obesity. With it, the body receives the substances necessary for the full work.

Keto Diet For Women

The recipe for effective and rapid weight loss within a month, or rather a week, begins to excite the population during the onset of the spring thaw. The gradual decrease in the number of outerwear makes you look more critically at your own body and the changes that have occurred during the winter months. The realization of the harm caused by the cold overtakes almost every woman. Therefore, to normalize weight and come to a more attractive appearance, a really effective diet for burning fat is suitable. One of the most popular for a month is a keto diet for women — the basic mechanisms of work, nutrition, and recipes that are sure to come in handy.

Basic Principles Of Nutrition On A Keto Diet

So, how does a keto diet work? To understand this, you will need to remember the physiology of nutrition. Whether it is male or female, the human body uses food as a fuel source for motor activity and creating reserves for a rainy day. Every day we eat foods that contain proteins, fats, and carbohydrates. The former is the building material for muscle tissue, the latter provide metabolic processes, and the third provides energy not only to the whole body but also to the brain.

If the carbohydrates in the woman's body are enough to ensure the body's stable functioning, its excess is processed into subcutaneous fat. This mechanism was available to mankind not out of harm but to ensure procreation because the existing surplus could at any moment turn into a deficit for a month. And the body needs a recipe to survive - using the accumulated stock.

The main principle of nutrition on a keto diet is a month's reduction to almost zero carbohydrate intake levels. As a result of this decision, the body will be forced to survive four main phases.

• The first phase of Keto: processing the last portion of carbohydrates within no more than 10 hours after a meal.

• The second phase of Keto: processing did not have time to be deposited in the form of a reserve of fat carbohydrates remaining in the liver.

• The third phase of Keto: the transition to alternative energy production from fats and proteins lasts from 3 to 8 days, or depending on the balance of nutrition, the intensity of training, and the body's fitness.

•	The fourth phase of Keto: the beginning of ketones' production - special substances that are obtained through the processing of subcutaneous fat and nourish the body with energy no worse than carbohydrates. As a result, a woman will need a little more than a week to switch to a weight loss regimen and then continue the diet until the moment when the weight comes to the ideal level.

The main sign of a complete transition to the state of processing fat in Keto is the appearance of energy and apathy's disappearance. Also, acetone's smell may appear in the mouth, which also indicates a transition to the regime of active weight loss. Improving the situation will help increased water consumption - up to four liters per day.

Many women compare recipes for a keto diet and a low carbohydrate diet but do not see the difference. The fact is that it consists of the number of harmful carbohydrates consumed per day.

For rational weight loss and not fasting, the body just needs fiber, which is found in vegetables. As a result of their own use in food, carbohydrates are also processed in parallel.

In a keto diet of only 30-50 grams per day, which is very small for a woman's body's normal functioning? And in a low carbohydrate diet, these components are more - up to 150 grams per day. This amount is enough to ensure the functioning of the brain. As a result, the body does not switch to ketone production like in Keto. Therefore, losing weight is also very rapid, but not as much as in the keto diet. But do not forget that a week is needed to switch to the regime.

Detailed Food Menu

So, as described above, the first week is for women a transition to a weight loss regimen. During this time, it will be essential to accurately calculate the protein and fat content in the diet to not experience stress and eat its own muscles with Keto. Therefore, the ratio of protein to fat will be either 50/50 or 60/40. This means that each ingredient consumed is decomposed into a complex content of 100 grams of the corresponding elements' product.

Important! A huge plus of the keto diet, many women, consider the lack of the need to reduce the daily diet by reducing calories. Weight loss occurs at 1200 Cal/day and 2500 Cal/day.

Another important point is the rejection of dairy products for effective weight loss. There is nothing harmful in them, but some milk substances can break down into carbohydrates, which will reduce a woman's chances to switch to a keto diet.

Now consider an approximate diet for a day.

• Breakfast: boiled egg - 2 pcs., Hard cheese 30 g, coffee - calorie content 290

Cal, protein / fat / carbohydrate ratio - 41 / 43.6 / 0.8

• Snack: almonds 30 g, calories 215 Cal, protein / fat / carbohydrate ratio - 6/19 / 5.4

• Lunch: 200 gr. Grilled breasts without oil, cucumber 100 gr., Calories 240 Cal, protein/fat/carbohydrate ratio - 48/4 / 3.7

• Snack: 150 gr steamed salmon, tomato 100 gr, calories 132 Cal, protein / fat / carbohydrate ratio - 40/22 / 3.8

• Dinner: cottage cheese 9% 150 gr, calorie content 255 Cal, protein / fat / carbohydrate ratio - 27/14 / 4,5

As you can see, only 18.2 g of carbohydrates per day with proper nutrition at 1132 Cal. This indicator is the minimum necessary. However, women can independently increase their caloric value by supplementing the diet with recipes from permitted foods and continue to lose weight - this is the beauty of Keto! The harm is that such a diet rarely causes a desire to eat more, as many foods are prohibited. Therefore, it is extremely difficult to withstand even the first week, especially a month.

Important! The principle of each diet is to achieve the desired result on the scales in a week or a month and the absence of harm. Therefore, a contraindication to Keto is diabetes - when ketones are produced, the condition worsens dramatically. Such a diet of Keto will also be harmful to women with diseases of the stomach and liver. A diet will also cause harm in the form of deterioration in brain activity and a decrease in reactions and concentration for intellectual workers. In addition, an unbalanced diet will require the intake of a vitamin-mineral complex. Therefore, it is worth assessing in advance the possible harm from Keto for a woman in order to mitigate the consequences.

Healthy Recipe

The secret of any keto diet recipe is to mix only foods that don't have carbohydrates but lots of protein and fat.

For example, a popular recipe for keto cheesecakes.

cottage cheese 9% 150 gr;

coconut flour 20 gr.;

one chicken egg.

Mix, portion, bake in the oven. Hearty but slightly dry cheesecakes will certainly be liked more if you add cinnamon or other seasonings to taste.

Ketogenic Diet: Lose Weight By Eating Fat

Mainly focused on fat consumption, this diet aims to minimize insulin production, the hormone responsible for storage. It upsets our eating habits and slimming reflexes. If it can boost an ad hoc basis, it cannot be followed in the long term without health risks.

The ketogenic diet was developed and used by different physicians in the early twentieth century to treat epilepsy. Abandoned when new drugs have emerged, it is prescribed again, mainly in pediatrics, children with epilepsy in whom treatments are ineffective or cause too many side effects.

Recently, scientists are interested in this diet for the management of overweight, type 2 diabetes, and even some cancers and neurological diseases. In Britain, recommended by nutritionists arrives in France, when carbohydrates (sugars), especially foods with a high glycemic index, are widely implicated in the epidemic of obesity.

What is the ketogenic diet?

The ketogenic diet is rich in lipids (fats), low in carbohydrates (sugars), and provides just the right amount of protein. This mode of food aims to minimize the release of insulin in the body, a hormone whose secretion is stimulated by the consumption of carbohydrates and promotes storage in fat cells. Without carbohydrates, the body is forced to produce ketone bodies from lipids to serve as an alternative fuel to the brain and the other organs, hence the term "ketogenic."

Keto Diet For Women Over 50

If you are a woman of 50 years or more and do not know what to do to lose weight, because here we bring you the solution, it is a diet based on the actual number of calories you should consume according to your age.

It is recommended to consume around 1,500 calories per day. However, if you are a sedentary woman, 1,200 calories per day are recommended. Remember that lack of physical activity increases the chances of gaining weight considerably.

The parts where fat is the most concentrated area, the hips, legs, and abdomen. Hormonal changes affect the body considerably. For this reason, for women of this age, their metabolism is slower, increasing the chances of gaining weight.

In general, the diet is requested to include:

1.   Fruits, vegetables, and legumes. The best source of protein is that which does not provide much fat, such as fish, chicken, turkey, and nuts.

2.   You should eat fat very sparingly and whenever they come from a healthy source, such as olive oil.

3.   To maintain healthy bones, you must take at least 1,200 mg of calcium a day. You can take it from food or take it in a supplement.

Primary sources of micronutrients:

•   With regard to dairy products, it is advisable to drink 1-2 glasses of skim milk or yogurt a day. One cup of yogurt contains about the same amount of calcium as 1 cup of milk.

•   It is also advisable to eat around 50 grams of fresh cheese.

•   To metabolize calcium, a sufficient amount of vitamin D is also needed, and women over 70 have to take a recommended daily dose of 800 IU. Sunlight helps get vitamin D, as do some foods, such as:

☐ Egg yolks

☐ The cheese

☐ Fortified dairy products.

☐ Ask your doctor concerning if a vitamin D supplement might be helpful.

☐ You may be interested: The best workout to burn belly fat.

In addition to this, it is recommended to take two and a half cups of vegetables a day — the more varied, the better. The diet of older women should be rich in fiber for the gastrointestinal organs to function correctly and avoid problems such as constipation.

Low carbohydrate and protein-rich diets are not very advisable for senior women, as they can cause metabolic problems.

It is best to eat mainly polyunsaturated and monounsaturated fat like the one that comes from olive oil, although you should not consume more than the equivalent of 5-6 teaspoons of oil a day.

Physical activity is good for burning the calories ingested, so it prevents weight gain. This doesn't mean that older people have to sign up for a gym or run a marathon.

Should Women Avoid The Keto Diet

Keto diet is now a diet trendy in the fitness community. It has become the best ally for weight loss and contributes to the reduction of intestinal inflammation at present. New research has shown positive effects for men and especially women who adhere to the keto weight loss diet.

Why is the Keto diet right for women?

The benefits of being a woman and following this diet are surprisingly good. In addition to weight loss and muscle gain, the female keto diet has a fantastic way to help the endocrine system, and as we all know, hormones have a significant effect on the whole body of a woman. Thus, hormones that fluctuate constantly can be responsible for pain, fatigue, and even depression. One can deny the relationship between hormones and cancer. A diet CETOS appears, thereby regulates the endocrine system by decreasing the incidence of certain cancers, thyroid disease, and diabetes.

Supportive research that supports the female keto diet.

It seems that the keto diet is sensitive to sex. To be sure: Researchers from the University of Iowa conducted a study to verify the effect in mice of a diet consisting of - 3% carbohydrates - 75% lipids, - 8% protein (against 47%, 7%, and 19% in a healthy diet).

Search results:

• It has been observed that the metabolism of females reacted less well than that of males. The work was presented at the end of March to the congress of the American Endocrinology Society.

• The female mice who were put on the keto diet had after 15 weeks, gained more weight than those not subjected to the ketogenic diet and controlled their blood sugar less well

• The males are under regime ketogenic them, had lost weight and fasting blood sugar in their blood was down compared to mice fed with a standard diet result, it follows that it is beautiful and well significant differences between men and women in terms of response to the ketogenic diet, which can be partially attributed to estrogen. The researchers who suspected estrogen were responsible for these differences; the authors repeated the protocol with females deprived of their ovaries. They then lost weight and fat mass under ketosis but still had trouble controlling their sugar levels. It is proven that postmenopausal women might get better weight loss with the ketosis diet. So the keto diet would be the diet for women 50 years older than most women. This is what was indicated: Jesse Cochran, the principal investigator. In a press release. The president of the Society of Endocrinology, E. Dale Abel, recommends above all to consult a doctor before following this type of diet

• For more annoying effects and the risk of weight regain after returning to a healthy diet, the ketogenic diet can cause deficiencies, high cholesterol, "foie gras," kidney stones, and osteoporosis.

How Does A Woman Initiate A Ketosis Diet?

- A ketogenic diet for women should not be started at 100%. You should slowly decrease the number of carbohydrates you consume slowly and carefully. -Avoiding carbs too quickly can have a negative effect; it can stress and confuse the body, causing a wild imbalance. - Caution should be doubled if you are pregnant or breastfeeding, need especially during this time; eat a balanced diet of fruits, fresh vegetables, dairy products, and cereals. In shod - L has dieters Keto is a regime Express for 50-year-old woman, according to this research, they are the most recommended to follow this weight loss diet.

- You must be careful to get a body as stable as possible, then slowly stir in the diet keto and mainly follow the recommendations of a nutritionist ketogenic diet.

The Ketogenic Diet In Practice

Authorized Foods, Prohibited Foods

In a balanced diet, carbohydrates provide about 50% of calories, fat, 35 to 40%, and protein 12 to 15%. In the ketogenic diet, lipids must represent at least 70% of energy intake and carbohydrates only 10%.

Specifically, you can eat all meats, including the most fat (lamb chop, pork loin, steak beef.), poultry with their skin, cold cuts, all fish including greasy fish (herring, mackerel, sardines, salmon), eggs, all cheeses, oleaginous fruits (avocado, olives, almonds, walnuts, hazelnuts, pistachios), tofu and tempeh (soy-based). The fat is used almost at will in seasoning or cooking. Butter, cream, or coconut oil is recommended daily because they are rich in "short and medium-chain fatty acids" that promote the process of ketosis (production of ketone bodies). Colza and nut oils are recommended for their essential Omega.

Aging Health And Ketosis

Aging brings about a certain decline in how we work, but that doesn't mean the process has to be isolating. Unfortunately, many seniors experience this differently.

A high-carbohydrate diet, with processed foods, often prescribed for people of this age group for convenience, can turn the aging process into something uncomfortable and debilitating.

However, you can support mental and physical health at any age through better nutrition. To answer our question at the beginning: yes, there are many benefits of a ketogenic diet for the elderly.

Benefits of A Ketogenic Diet

Here are some examples of problems that older people can face in their daily lives and the possibility of alleviating or even eliminating them by ketosis and eating healthy ketogenic foods:

Bone health: Osteoporosis, in which those bones become brittle and brittle, is one of the most common diseases in older men and women. Obtaining more calcium from daily dairy products, as is often recommended, is obviously not the answer. This can be the view from the fact that the countries with the highest rates of osteoporosis have the highest milk consumption. It is far better to focus on a ketogenic diet that contains little of the toxins that can affect absorption and is also rich in many micronutrients, rather than consuming too much of a certain micronutrient (calcium).

Inflammation: For many people, aging involves more Pain from injuries at a younger age or joint problems such as arthritis. Being in ketosis can assist reduce the production of cytokines that promote inflammation. This can help with such Pain and illness.

Insulin resistance: Some seniors in our society are overweight and need to be treated for insulin-related diseases, such as diabetes. This condition is serious as diabetes can lead to vision problems, kidney disease, and more. The ketogenic diet can definitely lead to a reduction in insulin resistance - the promotion of improved insulin sensitivity - and thus alleviate or even avoid diabetes.

Nutrient deficits: Older adults tend to have a greater lack of important nutrients such as

Vitamin D: The deficiency leads to cognitive impairments in older people, increases the risk of heart disease, and can even contribute to the risk of cancer

Vitamin B12: Insufficiency can lead to neurological diseases such as dementia.

Iron: The deficiency can lead to brain fog and fatigue

Fats: Lack of fats can lead to problems with perception, skin, eyesight, and vitamin deficiency.

The high-quality animal protein sources of the ketogenic diet can easily be excellent sources of these important nutrients.

Importance Of Ketosis For Aging

Ketogenic foods provide a high amount of nutrients per calorie. This is important because the basal metabolic rate (the number of calories needed to survive each day) is lower for older people, but they still need the same amount of nutrients as younger people.

A person aged 65 and over will find it much harder to make a living from junk food than a teenager or 20-year-old whose body is even more resilient. It is all the more important for seniors to eat foods that can support health and fight illnesses. This can make a significant difference - being able to enjoy life to the fullest or being in Pain and torturing.

Therefore, seniors have to eat an optimal diet by avoiding "empty calories" from sugar, for example, and improving their amount of nutrient-rich fats and proteins.

In addition, many of the foods selected by the elderly (or those that are administered in hospitals or clinical institutes) are often heavily processed and very low in nutrients — for example, white bread, pasta, mashed potatoes, pudding, etc.

It's pretty clear that the widespread high-carbohydrate diet isn't necessarily the best way to support seniors and their long-term health. A low-carbohydrate diet rich in animal and vegetable fats is far more positive for promoting better insulin sensitivity, preventing cognitive decline, and overall better health.

There is an interesting study in mice that examines how ketogenic diets can reduce middle-mortality and improve memory.

A ketogenic diet controls blood sugar.

As we discussed earlier, there is a link between high blood sugar and brain disorders such as Alzheimer's, dementia, and Parkinson's. Some factors that can contribute to Alzheimer's are:

Excessive intake of carbohydrates, especially sugar, which is drastically reduced in the ketogenic diet

Cell aging, which can be reduced by the ketogenic diet

Lack of dietary fats and cholesterol - these are plentiful and healthy in the ketogenic diet.

Using a ketogenic diet to control blood sugar and generally improve nutrition can help improve the insulin response and protect against memory problems that often occur with age.

The ketogenic diet for longevity

Regardless of your age, it is never a bad idea to improve your chances of feeling good and functioning optimally for the rest of your life. It is never too late to make improvements. The earlier we begin, the better our chances of preventing disease. Even for those who haven't treated the body for many years, as would have been appropriate, senior ketosis has the potential to repair some of the damage.

The earlier positive changes in diet that regulate healthy weight, blood sugar, immunity, and more, the greater the chance that you will later experience less Pain and illness and enjoy life better.

Reducing the amount of food in old age

Older people generally eat less. The lower intake of calories can easily lead to a reduction in energy if the metabolism is based on carbohydrates. In ketosis, the energy can remain more constant even if the person eats less.

It is important to have ketogenic-friendly snacks within reach at all times.

The Origin Of Ketogenic Diet

The ketogenic diet originated in the 20s in the medical field to treat cases of epilepsy.

Although this diet lost popularity for a time due to the development of new antiepileptic drugs, it gained fame for the treatment of refractory epilepsy (epilepsy that does not respond to antiepileptic drugs).

The diet consisted of a very high intake of fats, in a 4: 1 ratio to carbohydrates and proteins (i.e., four times more fat, by weight, than carbohydrates and proteins combined). In more specific numbers, the original ketogenic diet consisted of 1 g of protein per kg of body weight, no more than 15 g of carbohydrates per day, and the rest were fats.

This regimen helped patients (such as children) to control epileptic seizures that could not be controlled with traditional drugs.

Nowadays, however, many people follow the ketogenic diet not to treat epilepsy but to lose weight. And as a result, the current ketogenic diet has undergone some modifications concerning the original.

What exactly is gluconeogenesis?

When you are under a certain form of stress or when you consume an excess of proteins, your liver may use a process called gluconeogenesis to convert these proteins into glucose. If you dissect the word, then you can also deduce the meaning from this: 'gluco' naturally refers to glucose, 'neo' means 'new,' and 'genesis' means 'origin.'

Gluconeogenesis is one of the processes that take place in the liver that regulates blood sugar levels. This regulation depends on two peptide hormones: glucagon and insulin.

When you take a plate of sugared cornflakes and a glass of orange juice in the morning at breakfast, this is the signal for your pancreas to release insulin. The pancreas produces insulin and ends up in the blood that flows throughout the body.

There is a sort of 'lookout' for insulin on the outside of every cell of the body. As soon as the insulin passes into the bloodstream, it signals the cell so that the door opens to get blood sugar.

When insulin reaches the liver, it sends a signal here that the gluconeogenesis process must be stopped because there is enough glucose available in the blood. In addition, insulin acts as a signal that glucose must be stored in glycogen.

Insulin also encourages fat cells to store glucose as triglycerides and also inhibits the process of lipolysis. Lipolysis is the process by which fat molecules are broken down into glycerol and fatty acids.

When the body's cells have burned the sugars in the blood, the blood sugar level and with it also the insulin level in the blood drops, this is a sign for the pancreas to make the hormone glucagon.

Glucagon is, in a sense, the counterpart of insulin because it actually encourages the liver to restart the process of gluconeogenesis.

Because the glucagon level rises, the liver starts to break down glycogen (stored carbohydrates) and also breaks down proteins to form glucose (gluconeogenesis). At the same time, fat cells release their fatty acids into the blood, and lipolysis is encouraged.

One of the driving mechanisms behind the ketogenic diet and low carbohydrate diets, in general, is that insulin levels are lowered so that the body starts using glycogen and fat stores as an energy source.

By regulating insulin levels and minimizing carbohydrate intake, it is possible to make the transition from glycolysis (burning of sugars) to ketose (burning of fat).

During this transition, the body will first deplete the glycogen stores (glycogenolysis) and supply itself with glucose through gluconeogenesis.

The Transition From Glycolysis To Ketosis

The transition from glycogenolysis (glycogen as fuel) to gluconeogenesis (converting proteins into glucose as fuel) to eventual ketogenesis (converting fatty acids into ketones) can be explained in three phases that the human body goes through during a fasting period.

Phase 1: the post-absorbing phase (6 to 24 hours of fasting); during this phase, the body gets its energy from the supply of glycogen stored in the muscles and liver (glycogenolysis)

Phase 2: the gluconeogenic phase (2 to 10 days of fasting); during this phase, the glycogen supply is used up, and the body then switches to the gluconeogenesis process to provide energy. How long this phase takes depends on the person in question and, in particular, on the person's health.

Phase 3: the ketogenic phase (after ten days of fasting)

In this phase, the body switches to lipolysis, whereby fat is broken down into fatty acids and glycerol so that these can subsequently be converted into ketones and glucose, respectively.

Any person who switches from a carbohydrate-rich diet to a ketogenic diet will go through the above phases before they get into ketosis. It is important that you not only limit carbohydrate consumption but also moderate the number of proteins.

Ketogenic food does not mean that you mainly eat steak and eggs because then there is a good chance that you will get too many proteins.

This will keep your body in the gluconeogenic phase, where proteins are converted into glucose. With this, you will slow down the process of ketogenesis because the body still works on glucose.

Keto Diet and Menopause

Although technically, a woman reaches menopause after 12 months without a menstrual period, symptoms associated with perimenopause — the time onset of hormonal changes — can begin much earlier.

The average age at onset of perimenopause is 46 years and usually lasts about seven years. However, perimenopause can begin at any time between the mid-30s and mid-50s, and the transition can last from 4 to 14 years. The day after 12 months had passed without a menstrual cycle; it is considered already postmenopausal.

During and after the transition to menopause, up to 34 symptoms may appear. The most common ones are:

•   Night sweat

•   Weight gain, especially around the waist

- Insomnia

- Vaginal dryness

- Mood swings

- Fatigue

- Bad memory

Hormonal fluctuations and insulin resistance during menopause

During a woman's reproductive years, follicle-stimulating hormone (FSH) causes ovulation (the exit of an egg from a follicle) approximately every 28 days and stimulates ovarian estrogen production. After ovulation, the follicle in which the egg is placed produces progesterone.

However, when a woman enters perimenopause, her ovaries contain fewer eggs and produce less estrogen and progesterone. In response, the brain's pituitary gland enhances FSH production in an attempt to increase estrogen output. During this period, estrogen levels can fluctuate greatly, but they have been steadily declining over the past two years before menopause.

After puberty, estrogen typically routes fat to the hips. This is why many, though not all, women tend to gain weight in this area during their reproductive years.

However, as estrogen levels decrease during menopause, the fat storage goes to the stomach. Unlike subcutaneous fat stored on the hips, excess visceral fat affects not only your appearance and the size of your clothes. It is strongly associated with insulin resistance, heart disease, and other health problems.

Weight gain during menopause

In addition to changing the distribution of fat, most women note that their weight increases by several kilograms during and after perimenopause. This may seem to be due to a combination of several factors.

• First, lower estrogen levels contribute to insulin resistance and higher blood insulin levels or hyperinsulinemia, which contributes to weight gain.

• Secondly, studies show that in the early stages of perimenopause, the hunger hormone ghrelin levels increase.

Some women gain weight, even if they do not eat more than usual during menopause, due to hormonal changes.

Finally, the loss of muscle mass that occurs during menopause and the aging process can slow down metabolism, giving weight gain.

Low carbohydrate and keto diets to relieve menopause symptoms.

1. Weight Loss

A growing body of studies shows that low-carb diets and ketogenic diets are very effective for weight loss.

The main advantage of ketosis is the suppression of appetite, partially due to a decrease in ghrelin.

Indeed, a systematic review of 12 studies in 2014 found that a ketogenic diet reduces hunger and appetite. Moreover, the authors defined a ketogenic diet as one that produced fasting β-hydroxybutyrate levels in excess of or equal to 0.3 mm. This is actually a very mild ketosis level, which most people can achieve by limiting their intake of pure carbohydrates to 50 g or less per day.

2. Heat and fever

Unfortunately, there are currently no formal studies studying Keto's effects or low-carb diets on fever or fever.

However, many women who choose the catgo diet are seeing less and less intense tides. In some cases, the improvement seems quick and significant.

According to a retired neurosurgeon, Dr. Larry McCleury, there is a biochemical reason for this effect.

In his book The Brain Trust Program, Dr. McCleery explains that lowering estrogen during the menopausal transition reduces glucose transporters' effects for delivering glucose to the brain. He claims this process is similar to what happens in children with epilepsy and other seizures with seizures, although women in menopause experience this to a much lesser extent.

Dr. McCleury says women suffering from heart attacks can reduce their frequency and severity by following a low-carb diet that provides the brain with ketones, which are used as fuel. His dietary approach includes nutrients such as meat, fish, poultry, eggs, cheese, nuts, seeds, non-starchy vegetables, olive oil, and a small number of berries. In addition, he recommends fats, such as coconut oil or MCT oil, to naturally increase ketone levels.

3. Other symptoms of menopause

There are no studies to date that carbohydrate restriction has a positive effect on mood swings, brain clouding, irritability, and other mental or emotional changes characteristic of menopause.

However, some women during menopause reported that their mood, memory, and ability to concentrate improved as soon as they switched to a keto diet.

In addition, some studies show that keto foods can improve memory in older people with moderate cognitive deficits.

How many carbohydrates per day should a woman in menopause have?

Again, based on the lack of research in this area, it is difficult to formulate specific recommendations on women's number of carbohydrates during menopause. However, in general, limiting your intake to less than 50 g of pure carbohydrates per day will help suppress your appetite, lower your insulin levels and increase your sensitivity to insulin, which can help you lose weight.

Menopause Lifestyle

Physical activity

Staying active is vital during and after menopause. Researches in postmenopausal women have shown that regular exercise can help relieve stress, increase metabolism and fat burning, and prevent muscle loss. In addition, physical activity can potentially reduce heart attacks and fever.

One study discovered that women who participated in a six-month exercise program during menopause had lower rates of heart attacks than women who did not exercise.

Although all forms of exercise are useful, the most effective is strength training, which is used to treat the symptoms of menopause, slow down the aging process, and improve body composition.

In one study, 32 postmenopausal women conducted high-intensity workouts three times a week for 16 weeks, resulting in increased muscle strength, loss of abdomen, and a decrease in inflammatory processes.

Yoga

Yoga is well known for relieving stress. Several studies have found that yoga, tai chi, and similar mind-body treatments, can improve some of the symptoms of menopause, such as sleeping problems.

Moreover, yoga during menopause seems to enhance overall well-being and life satisfaction.

In a controlled study, 260 menopausal women who used yoga significantly improved their physical, psychological, and social quality of life.

Four Rules For Losing Weight After 50

Losing the weight gained as the age gets more difficult due to decreased movement and slowing down metabolism. However, with a few straightforward changes, you can get into the form in a short time.

1) Do weight or resistance exercises: The feature of these exercises is to load muscles in various ways and make them stronger. Of course, if you have never done these exercises before, it is useful to get approval from your doctor first.

2) Get enough protein: As the age gets older, consume protein suitable for your body weight as there is a decrease in muscle mass. The basic rule is to consume up to 1 g of protein per 1 kg of body weight. For example, if you are 70 kilos, the amount of protein you need to eat daily is 70 grams.

As for the amount of protein in food, one hundred grams of meat contain 30 grams, two eggs, 14 grams, and two matchboxes containing 10 grams of white cheese. Take the amount of protein daily by spreading it to meals, not just once. If you are looking for a practical method, this formula will be useful for you: Consume 15-20 g of protein in each main meal. If more is necessary, add protein to the snacks.

3) Don't be dehydrated: the body is dehydrated, you may feel hungry and eat more than you need. Take care to consume plenty of water, especially in the hot summer months. Your most important indicator of whether you drink enough fluids is your urine color. Make sure your urine is light yellow; the color darkening is a sign that you're not getting enough fluids.

4) Run your metabolism: The biggest mistake you make when you start a diet to lose weight is to implement a very low-calorie diet. As soon as you lower your daily calorie amount, your body will immediately slow down the metabolism to adapt to this situation. Pay more close attention to the quality of what you eat rather than calculate calories.

The simplest change you can make is to make sure that the foods you eat are the closest to nature, do not contain extra sugar, and do not bounce your blood sugar. You can consume vegetables, fruits, greens, nuts, and protein (such as meat, chicken, fish, eggs, cheese) without calculating calories and listening to your hunger.

Here Are Lists Of Keto Diet Recipes

1. Salmon and Spinach Rolls

Ingredients for Six Pieces

- Two eggs
- 200 g animal spinach (young spinach), 200g old Gouda
- 200 g smoked salmon, 100 g cream cheese
- Chives, dill
- Salt, pepper, nutmeg, Thaw spinach and express well.

Preparation

- Grind the cheese and mix with the eggs and the spinach to dough.
- Season it with a little salt, pepper, and nutmeg.
- Spread the dough on baking tray and bake at 200 degrees for about 20 minutes.

- Spread the cream cheese over the spinach dough and sprinkle with herbs.
- Spread the salmon slices thinly on the cream cheese. Leave a little 2 cm at the top.
- Roll the whole from below into a roll and cut into 2 cm wide rolls.

Tip: tastes warm as cold, preferably with a fresh herb quark dip and a fresh salad.

Nutritional Information per Piece:

- 315 kcal
- 25 g of fat
- 1 g carbohydrates
- 21 g protein

2. Pizza with Tuna Bottom

Ingredients for One Pizza Base

- One can of tuna in its juice
- One egg
- Salt pepper
- Thyme
- oregano

Preparation

- Tomato sauce, crème fraiche, cream cheese, savory spreads B. hemp spread the Mediterranean
- Tomatoes, peppers, mushrooms, olives, peppers, broccoli, rocket, spinach, red onions
- Mozzarella, Gouda, Feta
- Pine nuts, sunflower seeds, roasted almond sticks
- Preheat the oven to 220 ° C.
- Drain the tuna well, squeeze it with a fork in a bowl, and mix with the egg and then season with salt, pepper, and herbs.

- Spread out about 0.5 cm on a sheet of baking paper.
- Bake inside the oven for about 20-30 minutes, and then cover with the ingredients for the toppings and bake for another 5-10 minutes.

Nutritional Information per Piece of a pizza topped with vegetables and cheese:

- 641 kcal
- 44 g fat
- 11 g of carbohydrates
- 49 g of protein

3. Pumpkin stew with beef

Ingredients for Six Servings

- One small butternut squash
- 500 g beef goulash, 80 g of diced onion
- One diced carrot, 100 g of diced celery
- One diced garlic clove
- Three tablespoons butter, 3 tbsps. coconut oil
- Two tablespoons of flaxseed flour, and Salt pepper

Preparation

- Melt the butter, coconut oil and olive oil in a casserole dish and fry the meat all around. Add onion, carrot, and celery and fry briefly.
- Fill with water. Add flaxseed flour and garlic and stir well. Salts and peppers.
- Take the stew to a boil and simmer for 1-1.5 hours over medium heat.

- Preheat oven to 250 degrees. Divide the pumpkin, remove seeds, salt and pepper the two halves and roast in the oven for about 30-60 minutes, depending on size.
- Allow the pumpkin to cool slightly, cut into cubes and place in the stew just before the end of the cooking time.

Nutritional Information per Piece

- 312 kcal
- 20 g fat
- 10 g of carbohydrates
- 24 g protein

4. Crispy Chicken Thighs with Bacon

Ingredient

- Four chicken drumsticks (s)
- Eight slices/ s Bacon, about 100 g
- Herbs, Mediterranean (rosemary, thyme, oregano, lavender)
- sea salt
- 1 tbsp. olive oil

Cooking time: approx. 50 min

Calorie: about 300 kcal

Preparation

- Preheat oven at 180 ° C (160 ° C convection). Wash the chicken thighs and pat dry.
- Heat up the olive oil inside a frying pan (if oven suitable) and fry the legs from all sides. Remove from the pan, season well all around (freshly chopped Mediterranean herbs or a high-quality dry mix) and salt. Then

wrap with two slices of bacon, if necessary fix with wooden toothpicks, roast again in the still hot pan from above and below. Be careful when turning.

- Put the pan inside the oven for 30 minutes and add a touch of olive oil if necessary. If there is no pan suitable for cooking, place the legs on the oven rack and push a sheet of baking paper under it as a safety catch, after half the time turn the thighs. Serve hot!

It fits a light raw food salad.

Tip:

Do not use a casserole dish (used in the photo only for decorative purposes). In this, the thighs swim too much in their juice and are therefore not crispy.

Nutritional Information per Piece
- 300 kcal
- 16 g fat (of which 6 g total fat)
- KH 600 mg
- Protein 40 g

5. Cucumber salad

Preparation time: 10 minutes

Total time: 10 minutes

Ingredients

1 small red onion, sliced into thin slices

2 cucumbers, peeled or not (depending on the variety of cucumber and its taste), and cut into thin slices

Juice of 2-3 medium lemons

2 tablespoons chopped coriander finely (you can also use parsley)

2 tablespoons of olive oil

Salt to taste

Preparation

1. Put the onion slices in a dish and sprinkle with half a tablespoon of salt. Rub the onions with the salt and

then cover them with water for a few minutes. Then sift and rinse the onions well. This helps to remove the bitter and strong flavor of the onions.

2. Mix cucumber slices, washed onion, lemon juice, chopped coriander, and olive oil.3Mix well and then adjust the salt to taste.

3. The salad can be served immediately, or it can be left to rest for at least 30 minutes before serving.

Nutrition

Net carbohydrates: 3% (6 g)

Fiber: 5 g

Fat: 79% (67 g)

Protein: 18% (35 g)

kcal: 774

6. Corn salad, potatoes, and broccoli

Yield: For 2

Ingredients

1 cups corn kernels or fresh corn, almost 4 ears of corn, steamed or boiled

2 cups cooked potatoes, diced, about 3 medium potatoes

2 cups of broccoli flowers, lightly steamed or boiled

½ cup finely chopped red onion

2 tablespoons mayonnaise (you can also use plain yogurt)

1 garlic cloves, crushed

1 tablespoons coriander or finely chopped cilantro

1 tablespoons of lemon juice

½ teaspoon of wasabi pasta (or you can use horseradish / spicy mustard), fit to taste

Salt and pepper to taste

Preparation

- To prepare the dressing, combine the mayonnaise, crushed garlic, chopped coriander, lemon juice, wasabi paste, salt, and pepper inside a small bowl and then mix well.
- In a large salad bowl, add corn or fresh corn, potatoes, broccoli, and chopped onion.
- Add mayonnaise dressing with wasabi, mix well and serve immediately or refrigerate until meal time.

Nutrition

Energy   1480kj

Carbohydrates: 4% (7 g)

Fiber: 3 g

Fat: 77% (57 g)

Protein: 19% (32 g)

kcal: 674

7. Italian keto meatballs with mozzarella cheese

Tomato sauce, rich and comforting. Mozzarella, fresh and creamy. Meatballs, with the right touch of onion and oregano. It's like eating spaghetti, but without carbohydrates. Enjoy every bite, ketolicious!

Ingredients

450 g ground beef

50 g grated Parmesan cheese

1 egg

½ tbsp. dried basil

½ tsp. ground onion

1 tsp. garlic powder

1 tsp. Salt

½ tsp. ground black pepper

3 tbsps. olive oil

400 g canned whole tomatoes

2 tbsps. fresh parsley, finely chopped

200 g fresh spinach

50 g butter

150 g (325 ml) fresh mozzarella cheese

Salt and pepper

Preparation

Place the ground beef, Parmesan cheese, eggs, salt and spices in a bowl and mix well. Assemble the meatballs with the mixture, approximately 30 grams (1 ounce) each. It is easier if you keep your hands moist while you make the meatballs.

Heat the olive oil inside a large pan and sauté the meatballs until golden brown on all sides.

Reduce heat and add canned tomatoes. Let it simmer for 17 minutes, stirring every couple of minutes. Salpimentar to taste. Add the parsley and stir. You can prepare the dish here to freeze it.

Melt the butter in another pan and fry the spinach for 1-2 minutes, stirring continuously. Salpimentar to taste. Add spinach to meatballs. Cover with fresh mozzarella cheese, cut into bite-sized pieces. Serve and enjoy.

Nutrition

Low carb ketogenic

Per portion

Net carbohydrates: 3% (5 g)

Fiber: 3 g

Fat: 72% (50 g)

Protein: 25% (39 g)

kcal: 628

8. Ketogenic Frittata with mushrooms and cheese

They are also known as "the open omelet of Italy". Frittatas are easy to prepare and super versatile, you can enjoy them at any time of the day. This version contains fresh mushrooms and cream cheese: They are the perfect complement for eggs in this classic ketogenic dish.

Ingredients

Frittata

450 g mushrooms

90 g butter

6 scallions

1 tbsp. fresh parsley

1 tsp. Salt

½ tsp. ground black pepper

10 eggs

225 g grated cheese

240 ml (225 g) mayonnaise

110 g green leafy vegetables

Preparation

Preheat your oven temperature to 175 ° C (350 ° F). First, prepare the vinaigrette sauce and set aside.

Cut the mushrooms in the shape and size you want.

Sauté mushrooms over medium heat in most butter until golden brown. Lower the heat. Save some butter to grease the roasting pan.

Chop up the scallions and then mix them with the fried mushrooms. Add salt and pepper then mix with parsley.

Mix the eggs, mayonnaise and then cheese in a separate bowl. Salpimentar to taste.

Add the mushrooms and the scallions and pour everything in a well-greased roasting pan. Bake for 30-40 mins or until the frittata turns golden brown and the eggs are cooked.

Allow it cool for 10 minutes and then serve with green leafy vegetables and vinaigrette sauce.

Nutrition

Per portion

Net carbohydrates: 2% (6 g)

Fiber: 2 g

Fat: 84% (87 g)

Protein: 14% (32 g)

kcal: 934

9. Maria's keto pancakes

Pancakes for dinner? Why not... Prepared in minutes and very satiating, these ketogenic delights go well with any meal. So put the pan on the fire and cook!

Ingredients

20 g pork rinds

2 eggs

2 tbsps. unsweetened cashew milk

1 tsp. maple extract

1 tsp. ground cinnamon

2 tbsps. (25 g) coconut oil, for frying

Preparation

Place the pork rinds inside a blender and press until they are made fine powder. Add the remains of the ingredients and mix until uniform.

Heat a pan over medium heat; when it's hot, add a tablespoon of coconut oil.

Pour ¼ cup of the mixture in the pan. Fry until golden brown and set aside, about 2 minutes. Flip and continue cooking until it is completely done.

Remove from the pan and then repeat with the remaining dough. Add more coconut oil if necessary.

Nutrition

Low carb ketogenic

Per portion

Fiber: 1 g

Fat: 79% (42 g)

Protein: 20% (24 g)

Kcal: 499

10. Keto bacon and eggs dish.

Do not cut yourself and enjoy this classic ketogenic breakfast for lunch. Or dinner. We have added nuts and peppers to make it crispy. Why complicate things?

Ingredients

150 g bacon

2 tbsps. butter, for frying

4 eggs

2 avocados

4 tbsps. (25 g) nuts

1 green paprika

Salt and pepper

1 tbsp. fresh chives, finely chopped (optional)

At your service

30 g arugula

2 tbsp olive oil

Preparation

Fry bacon inside butter over medium heat till its crispy.

Remove from pan and keep warm. Leave the accumulated fat in the pan. Reduce the heat to medium and then fry the eggs in the same pan.

Place the bacon, eggs, avocado, nuts, pepper and arugula on a plate.

Pour the remaining bacon fat over the eggs. Season to taste.

Nutrition

Low carb ketogenic

Per portion

Net carbohydrates: 3% (8 g)

Fiber: 16 g

Fat: 86% (100 g)

Protein: 10% (27 g)

kcal: 1066

11. Tofu and broccoli salad

- Sauce
- ½ cup (125 mL) water
- 125 ml (½ cup) of hoisin sauce
- 1 cinnamon stick
- 4 star anis
- Jumped up
- 454 g (1 lb.) firm tofu, diced
- ¼ cup (60 mL) canola oil
- 1 broccoli, cut into small bunches
- 1 onion, finely chopped
- 2 cloves of garlic, chopped
- 1/3 cup (75 mL) unsalted peanuts, toasted and crushed

Preparation

- Sauce
- Inside a saucepan, take it to the boil all the ingredients. Simmer it for about 3 minutes or till the sauce is slightly syrupy. Remove the spices.
- Jumped up

In a pan, brown the tofu in the oil. Add broccoli and then cook for about 5 minutes on medium heat or until broccoli is al dente. Put onion and the garlic and sauté for 2 minutes. Add the sauce and mix well. Continue cooking for about 2 minutes. Serve on rice vermicelli. Garnish with peanuts.

12. Pumpkin and apple soup

Ingredients

- 450 grams (1 lb.) pumpkin
- 1 Granny Smith apple cored, and quartered
- One medium onion cut
- Two cloves garlic
- One tablespoon of olive oil
- salt
- ¼ teaspoon of cayenne more to taste
- 300 ml (1¼ cup) of vegetable stock
- freshly ground black pepper to add taste

- GARNISH:
- pomegranate arils

- some pumpkin seeds
- fresh parsley finely chopped

Preparation

- Preheat the oven about 200 degrees C (or 392 degrees F). Line a large baking sheet with a parchment paper.
- Cut the pumpkin half lengthways and scoop out seeds.
- Slice each pumpkin half in half to make quarters and place, cut-side up, on a baking tray, along with the onions.
- Drizzle with olive oil and then sprinkle some salt.
- Bake for about 20 minutes, then add the garlic and apple, flip the pumpkin cut side down and then roast for another for 20 minutes, or until the flesh is soft.
- Use a spoon to scoop out the flesh of the pumpkin and transfer to a high-speed blender with the apple, onion, garlic (remove the skins), cayenne, and vegetable stock.
- Blend on high for almost 2 minutes, or until silky smooth.

- If too thick, add vegetable stock to thin it out and blend over. Taste and adjust the seasonings.
- Serve, ladle soup into a bowl, and with pomegranate arils, pumpkin seeds, fresh parsley and freshly ground black pepper.
- Then serve.
- Refrigerate it leftovers in an airtight container for 4 days.

13. Tuna fillets with all tomatoes salad

Ingredients

- 4 Tuna steaks without skin.
- 2 Tablespoons of extra virgin olive oil.
- 1 Shallot medium, finely chopped.
- 180 grs. of yellow and red cherry tomatoes mixed, cut in half.
- 50 grs. Of green olives without bone, sliced.
- 2 Tablespoons fresh basil, finely chopped.
- ½ Tablespoon of lemon juice.

- Sea salt and freshly ground black pepper.

Preparation

- Season the tuna steaks with one teaspoon of salt and ¼ tablespoon of pepper. Heat the oil in a large Magefesa Skillet over medium-high heat. Place the tuna in the pan in a single layer and cook, turning once, until it is made based on your preferences. Estimate about 3 or 4 minutes on average. Transfer the tuna to a large dish and reserve.
- Reduce to medium heat and add the shallot to the pan. Cook, stirring, until golden brown, about 1 minute. Add the tomatoes, olives, basil, ½ teaspoon of salt, and a pinch of ground pepper. Cook until the tomatoes begin to acquire a smooth texture, about 2 minutes more. Take out the pan from the heat and then slowly add the lemon juice. Pour the tomato salad over the reserved tuna steaks and serve.

14. Asparagus and green pea's salad

Ingredients

- 1/2 of bunch (8 ounces) asparagus
- 1 1/2 cups of shelled English peas, blanched
- 1/4 cup of fresh mint leaves (you can tear it, if large)
- 1/4 cup of chopped toasted almonds, plus more for serving
- Two tablespoons extra-virgin olive oil
- Two tablespoons of rice-wine vinegar
- Kosher salt and freshly ground pepper

Preparation

1. Trim asparagus. Thinly slice on a strong bias. Toss with peas, mint, almonds, oil, and vinegar. Season with salt and then add pepper, and serve, topped with more mint and almonds.

22. Reds salad on bacon and balsamic vinaigrette

Ingredients

- Balsamic vinaigrette:
- ¼ cup olive oil
- Three tablespoons balsamic vinegar
- ½ teaspoon finely chopped garlic
- ¾ Dijon mustard spoon
- ¾ honey bee teaspoon
- Salt and pepper to taste
- Salad with red grapes, bacon, and walnut:
- 3 cups mixed lettuce (escarole, French, ball, Italian)
- ½ cup red grapes, in halves
- Two slices of bacon, golden brown
- 8-10 praline or natural walnuts
- Two tablespoons blue cheese, Roquefort or blue cheese

Preparation

- Balsamic vinegar vinaigrette:
- Mix all ingredients in a jar, cup or dish and mix well until everything is well incorporated.

- Add season to taste.
- Salad with red grapes:
- Cook the bacon until well browned and cut into medium pieces.
- Mix the lettuce with half of the balsamic vinaigrette.
- Place on a plate.
- Add the red grapes in halves, the bacon in pieces, the blue cheese, and the nuts.
- Serve with the remaining vinaigrette.

23. Arugula, lettuce and strawberry salad

Ingredients

- ¼ red onion, thinly sliced
- 4 cups of arugula leaves
- 250 g tapered strawberries
- 90 g goat cheese crumbled
- 1 to 2 cases of balsamic vinegar
- 2 to 3 cases of olive oil
- The salt according to your taste

Preparation

- Dip the onions in cold, lightly salted water to remove the bitter side.
- Mix the balsamic vinegar, olive oil and salt in a tight container and shake to the rhythm of the salsa.
- Drain the onions and mix with the arugula leaves and the vinaigrette.
- Top with crumbled cheese, sliced strawberries, and spicy pecans.
- Mix at the table and serve immediately.

24. Curry tuna salad

Ingredients

- 400 g natural tuna one beautiful romaine 100 g raisins two medium pippin apples one lemon juice one teaspoon curry 1 cup mayonnaise

Preparation of the tuna salad with curry:

- Open the can of tuna. Drain and divide into large pieces.

- Wash and dry the salad leaves thoroughly. Peel apples before cutting into thin slices sprinkle the lemon juice to prevent them from turning black.
- Dressing the tuna salad with curry:
- In a salad bowl, arrange the salad leaves, the pieces of tuna, the raisins and the slices of apple to mix everything.
- Add the curry to the mayonnaise and stir well.
- Mix the mayonnaise with the salad just before serving.

25. Beets cucumber salad with curry vinaigrette

Ingredients:

- QS beetroot
- QS of apples
- QS chicken breast
- Classic curry vinaigrette
- nuts and nuts
- salt and freshly ground pepper

Preparation:

- Salt the chicken breasts and cook in a drizzle of oil. Book them 5 minutes.
- Peel the beets, and grate them with a robot or julienne with a mandolin.
- Cut the apples into fine julienne with a mandolin or knife, or dice to make it easier. You can peel them first Reserve the julienne or the dice in the refrigerator.
- Prepare classic vinaigrette by adding curry powder, and season the beets.
- Arrange the beets on the plate add the diced apples or julienne and crushed hazelnuts.
- Slice or dice the chicken breasts and add them to the beets.
- It's ready to eat.

26. Roasted carrots and cashew salad on lemon vinaigrette

Ingredients / for 2 people

- Four beautiful carrots
- One wrist of cashew nuts
- One wrist of parsley or coriander
- One tablespoon soup grape dry
- For seasoning:
- One lemon
- One tablespoon of tahini
- Two tablespoons of olive oil
- One tablespoon of hazelnut oil

Preparation

- 1 Peel the carrots and grate them. Put them on a serving plate. Mince the parsley and add to the carrots. Add the raisins on top.
- 2 Heat 1 tablespoon of vegetable oil in a skillet over high heat and sauté the cashews. Stir frequently, so they do not burn. When they turn a beautiful golden color, place them on paper towels and salt them. Let

itcool before you add them to the carrots.

- 3 Prepare the seasoning: squeeze the lemon and place the juice in a bowl. Add the tablespoon tahini and mix well with a fork to fully dilute the sesame puree. Add two tablespoons of olive oil with a tablespoon of hazelnut oil. Mix the sauce well to incorporate the oils.

27. Baby spinach, chicken and carrot salad with red wine dressing

Ingredients

- Carrots: 2
- Red onions: 3
- Spinach sprouts: 80 g
- Olive oil: 3 tbsp. soup
- Lemon juice: 0.5 tbsp. coffee
- Juice of 1/2 orange
- Agave syrup: 1 tbsp. coffee

Preparation

- Peel the carrots and onions. Cut the carrots into slices using a thrifty knife and sliced onions.
- Wash the spinach sprouts, and then drain them. Mix in a medium bowl with the carrots and onions.
- Mix the agave syrup with the olive oil and the orange and lemon juice. Pour over the salad and mix before serving. Enjoy it immediately.

28. Plum tomatoes and peppers salad

Ingredients

- Green peppers: 2
- Red peppers: 2
- Yellow peppers: 2
- Cherry tomatoes: 400 g
- Yellow lemon: 1
- Olive oil: 5 cl
- Bouquet of parsley dish: 1
- Red onion: 1
- Salt
- Pepper

Preparation

- Take off the first skin of your bunion and chisel it.
- Wash your peppers. Cut them in 2, eliminate the peduncles, the seeds as well as the white dimensions. Cut the flesh into small cubes.
- Wash and cut your cherry tomatoes in 2 or quarters according to their sizes.
- In a salad bowl, mix the tomatoes with the peppers, the onion, the juice of your lemon, the olive oil, salt, and pepper.
- Chop the parsley.
- Serve your salad by garnish with parsley.

29. Spinach and avocado with quail eggs

Ingredients:

- One quail eggs
- Two rocket lettuce
- Two spinach
- One watercress
- One red onion
- Two avocado

- Three pecan nuts
- One tablespoon of olive oil
- One fresh ground pepper

Preparations

Good QUAIL EGGS:

- TO SOFT BOIL IT: place it in gently boiling water for about 1 minute, leave eggs into the water for a further 30 seconds, remove it and then peel the shells then serve.
- TO HARD BOIL: place it gently into the boiling water for about 2 1/2 minutes, remove, run under cold water, then peel the shells and serve.

30. Eggplant and pine nuts salad

Ingredients For the salad are

- One tablespoon of coriander seeds
- One teaspoon of cumin seeds

- Two eggplants of (aubergines), peeled and cut into large chunks
- Two tablespoons of oil, plus extra for frying
- Two garlic of cloves
- gluten-free flour, for dusting
- ⅔ cup (3½ oz/100 g) pine nuts
- One bunch parsley leaves coarsely well chopped
- a handful of baby spinach leaves, chopped
- a handful of pomegranate seeds
- salt and pepper
- For the dressing
- Four tablespoons pomegranate juice
- One teaspoon balsamic vinegar
- juice ½ lemon
- Four tablespoons of olive oil
- salt and pepper

Preparation

- Preheat the oven to about 200 ° C gases.
- Put the coriander and cumin seeds in a deep mortar and then crush them with a pestle. Toast them into a dry skillet or frying pan for a few minutes, or until fragrant.

- Put the eggplants (aubergines) in a large bowl and toss with olive oil, crushed garlic, salt, and with pepper then sprinkle on the toasted coriander and cumin seeds.
- Drizzle one tablespoon of oil onto a baking sheet. Then dip the eggplants lightly in the flour. Place them all inside the baking sheet and then roast for 30 minutes, or until chargrilled and slightly crisp. Let cool.
- While the eggplants are there roasting, mix all the dressing ingredients and set aside.
- Put the roasted eggplants into a medium bowl, pour 1–2 tablespoons of the dressing, and toss well. Let stand for about 10 minutes so that the dressing can be absorbed.
- Heat 2 teaspoons of olive oil into a skillet and lightly toast the pine nuts until it appears golden.
- Add the chopped parsley, spinach, and then pomegranate seeds to the eggplants and toss them all together well. Sprinkle the toasted pine nuts and serve with the remaining dressing.

31. Ripe tomatoes and basil salad

Ingredients

Serves: 2

- Four vines ripened tomatoes
- good pinch sea salt
- handful basil leaves rolled and thinly sliced
- One tablespoon good aged balsamic vinegar
- One tablespoon extra-virgin olive oil

Preparation

- Prep: 5min
- Ready in 5min
- Grab an attractive serving plate; flat glass or black works nicely. Slice the tomatoes thinly and scatter onto a plate. Sprinkle with salt, then spread all over the basil leaves. Drizzle over the vinegar and oil. Cover with cling film and then leave at room temperature until ready to serve.

32. Mango, kiwi and berries salad

Ingredients

- Two lemons, juiced
- One teaspoon honey
- Two tablespoons chopped fresh mint, + extra leaves for garnish
- 1 pound mango chunks
- 1 pound kiwis, peeled and sliced
- 1 pound strawberries, hulled and quartered
- Preparation
- In the small bowl, whisk together the lemon juice, honey, and chopped fresh mint. Set aside while preparing the fruit to allow the mint to infuse the mixture. You can make this up to one day ahead.
- Put the fruit pieces in the large bowl and gently toss with the lemon mixture. Chill in the refrigerator until its ready to be served. Best eaten within a few hours.

33. Bulgur, cucumber and orange salad

Ingredients

- 1/3 cup of uncooked bulgur
- One large orange, peeled and well chopped (3/4 cup)
- One medium onion, chopped (1/2 cup)
- One small tomato, chopped (1/2 cup)
- 3/4 cup of chopped fresh parsley
- Two tablespoons of lemon juice
- Two teaspoons of grated orange peel
- Two teaspoons of olive or vegetable oil
- 1/2 teaspoon of salt
- 1/4
- teaspoon pepper
- 1/8
- teaspoon crushed red pepper flakes

Preparation

- 1 Cooked bulgur. In the glass, toss bulgur and all remaining ingredients.

- 2 Cover it and then refrigerate it for about 2 hours or until chilled.

34. Cucumber, lettuce and crabmeat salad

Ingredients for Crab Salad:

- 1 lb. (16 oz.) package Imitation crab meat, chopped up into a small pieces
- 1 English One long cucumber, diced small
- Two medium tomatoes, diced and drained any excess juice
- 1/4 cup of chopped Green onions, fresh or frozen
- Three cloves of garlic
- 1/2 cup of mayo, or to taste (I'm keeping it healthier with a vegenaise)

Preparation

Crab Salad:

- Chop crab into small pieces. Chop with knife or use a food processor and pulse in batches. Shred it apart a little for a nice coating.

- Chop two medium tomatoes and drained them of excess juice. Seed to keep the salad from getting juicy the next day make small dice out of the cucumber. In a bowl, combine chopped tomatoes, diced cucumbers; shredded crab and 1/4 cup diced green onion.
- In a small bowl, combine with 1/2 cup mayo and three pressed cloves of garlic. Add the dressing to the crab salad for taste. You can add more mayo if you like a juicier salad. Refrigerate until it's ready to serve.

35. Creamy chicken, grapes and chestnuts salad

Ingredients

- 1 cup of real mayonnaise
- 1 8 of oz. package cream cheese, softened
- One tablespoon of season salt

- 3 cups of cooked and cubed chicken
- 3 cups of chopped celery
- 3 cups of red or green seedless grapes halved
- One small can of water chestnuts drained
- 3/4 cup of chopped green onions
- 1/2 cup of chopped bell pepper
- Toasted almonds for garnishing
- Bread of choice

Preparation

- In a bowl combine the mayonnaise, with cream cheese, and season salt. Add in the remaining part of the ingredients except for the almonds and gently combine.
- Serve immediately as a salad or sandwich--or make in advance (tastes even better the next day.)

36. Cauliflower, carrots and peas curry

Ingredients:

- 40 grams of cooked cauliflower
- 1 cup of frozen peas
- Three units of tomato
- Four units of Ajetes
- One pinch of salt
- One pinch of ground black pepper
- One tablespoon dessert curry powder
- One carrot unit
- One handful of fresh Cilantro
- 100 milliliters of water
- Three tablespoons of olive oil

Preparation

- Gather all the ingredients to make the pea and tomato curry. This recipe is also very good with vegetables such as zucchini or broccoli.
- Clean the young garlic by removing the green end and the lower part of the stems. Cut them as indicated in

the image and sauté them in a pan with olive oil for a couple of minutes.

- Peel the carrots, and then cut it into slices and add it to the pan. Let cook for 3 minutes.
- Next, add the tomato peeled and cut into squares. Add a little salt and ground pepper, let cook for 5 minutes.
- At this moment incorporate the curry. I have used a prepared mixture of spices for curry, similar to the great masala.
- It is necessary that the curry is cooked with the rest of the ingredients for a couple of minutes over medium heat. After that time add the water and let it boil for another 3 minutes.
- Add the frozen peas and get them to boil with the remaining ingredients for 2 minutes.
- Finally, add the cooked cauliflower and let it mix well with the chickpea and tomato curry. The cauliflower makes the dish more consistent and gives us potassium and calcium.

- Serve the vegan curry of peas and tomato with basmati rice or jasmine rice. If you are thinking of other recipes with curry you can try the green curry with prawns or the quinoa curry. Hope you like it.

37. Halibut with orange and broccoli

Ingredients

- 4 halibut fillets (200 gr each)
- 3 teaspoons of fish stock
- 2 broccoli
- 4 tablespoons olive oil
- 60 cl of cream
- 7 branches of fresh tarragon
- 10 cl white wine "Bordeaux" dry (Entre-Deux-Mers)
- Maïzena express
- Pepper
- Salt
- Garlic
- Nutmeg
- 3 Oranges

Preparations

- In a dish, put olive oil with salt, pepper and garlic powder. To mix everything.
- Add the halibut fillets by brushing them with the mixture.
- Before cooking halibut fillets, cut, clean and make small bunches of broccoli.
- Steam them for 25 minutes.
- Preheat oven 5 min. at 180 ° and put in the halibut fillets. Cook for 20 minutes at 180 °.
- During this time, finely cut the leaves of tarragon.
- In a bowl, mix the cream and the fish stock. Then add the finely chopped tarragon, salt and pepper and mix everything together.
- In a skillet, heat the sauce by adding the white wine and the juice of a orange.
- Make thicken with the maizena to obtain a smooth sauce.
- Squeeze the remaining 2 oranges, add a little salt, pepper and nutmeg and sprinkle the broccoli when they are cooked.

38. Chicken fillet soup

Ingredients

- 600 g of chicken fillet
- 3 or 4 carrots
- 1 celery stalk
- 3 onions
- 2 cloves garlic
- 1 C. butter
- 1 liter of water
- 50 cl l of milk
- 40 g corn flour
- 2 cubes of chicken broth
- 4 c. dehydrated poultry ground coffee
- Salt pepper

Preparation

- Wash onions and garlic. Chop the onions and chop the garlic.
- Peel off the carrots and the celery and cut them into small cubes.
- Cut the chicken fillets into thin slices, and then set aside.
- In a casserole dish or use a large saucepan, melt the butter and add the

onions that you will return to medium heat until they are a little golden.

- After a few minutes, add chopped garlic, diced carrots and celery, and chicken slices. Salt a little and pepper.
- Sauté for some minutes over medium heat until chicken is golden brown.

39. Mackerel steaks in butter

Ingredients

- Bunch of dill: 1
- Onions (small): 2
- Oil: 2 tbsp. soup
- Lemon juice: 2
- Salt
- Pepper
- For lemon butter:
- Butter: 200 g
- Lemon juice: 2
- Fresh cream: 10 cl
- Salt
- Cayenne pepper

Preparation

- Empty, cut and clean the fish by your fishmonger. Peel the onions and cut them into thin slices; wash the dill. Season the inside part of the fish and add the dill sprigs.
- Preheat the oven to 240 ° C. Cut 4 rectangles of parchment paper (about 22 x 24 cm). Place on each a few slices of onions then add the mackerel, incise their skin; sprinkle with olive oil and lemon juice. Close the wrappers tightly while rolling the edges.
- Prepare the lemon butter: put the cream in a saucepan and reduce to 2/3; add the butter gradually in small pieces. Stir with a whisk over a very soft fire. Top with lemon juice and season with salt and cayenne pepper; keep the sauce warm in a bain-marie.
- Put the wrappers on a plate and cook them in the oven for 8 minutes. Serve the wrappers directly on a plate and let the guests open them themselves to smell the cooking fragrance.

40. Tart apple and carrots soup

Ingredients

- 800 g carrots
- 2 golden apples
- 1 onion
- 1.5 liters of water
- 1 cubic broth of vegetables preferably
- Ginger
- Salt pepper

Preparation

- Wash and peel the carrots and apples, cut into small pieces.
- Cut the onion and sweat it in a pan with oil.
- Add carrots and apples.
- In a saucepan, melt the cubed vegetable broth in 1.5 liters of water.
- Cover the vegetables with the broth.
- Season and boil for 30 minutes.
- Mix everything together.

41. Black bean and avocado soup

Ingredients

Servings: 10

- 1 can (540 ml) of black beans, well drained
- 1 can (398 ml) corn kernels, drained
- 4 Roma tomatoes, seeded and chopped
- 1 red pepper, diced
- 1 jalapeno pepper, chopped
- 1/3 cup chopped fresh cilantro
- 1/4 cup red onion
- 1/4 cup fresh lime juice
- 2 tbsp. red wine vinegar
- 1 C. salt
- 1/2 c. pepper
- 2 lawyers, diced

Preparations

- Add all ingredients except avocados inside a large bowl and mix. Add the avocados and mix gently. Cover with plastic wrap (directly on the salsa) and refrigerate at least 2 hours before serving.

42. Zucchini and shrimps salad

Ingredients

- 1 zucchini
- 1 small shrimp box
- 1 lemon
- 3 tablespoons of oil
- 1 tablespoon of vinegar
- Pepper
- Salt

Preparation

- Grate the zucchini in julienne and rinse the shrimps in clear water then mix zucchini and shrimps in a salad bowl.
- Prepare the vinaigrette with the oil, vinegar, salt and pepper.
- To water the salad.
- Take more or less fine zest on the lemon and incorporate in the salad.
- That's ready, you just have to feast.

43. Creamy and cheesy aubergine

Ingredients

- 4 beautiful aubergines
- 50 g of fromage frais
- 1/2 teaspoon garlic powder
- 6 tablespoons of olive oil
- Salt to taste

Preparations

- Wash the aubergines carefully and place them on a baking sheet lined with parchment paper. The paper is very important because the juice comes out of the eggplant and caramelizes in the oven and then attaches a lot, the paper avoids that.
- Put in the oven at 240 ° C (tea 8) for 1 hour by turning the aubergines halfway through cooking. They must burn a little to give the smoked taste. Split the eggplant in half lengthwise and hollow out with a spoon scraping the pulp, closer to the skin.
- Pour the pulp of the aubergines removed from the skin in a blender.

- Add half a teaspoon of garlic powder including the fresh cheese and put the mixer on the road.
- While the mixer turns for olive oil and a little salt.
- After having tasted and possibly rectified in salt, pour in a dish the eggplant caviar and decorate with green olives cut in half. Keep in cool until serving.

44. Pressure cooked mixed vegetables

Ingredients

- 500 g Carrot (s), peeled, cut into 1cm slices
- 60 g   Herb butter
- 250 g Peas, TK
- Salt
- Pepper
- 1 1 / 2 EL sugar
- 1 / 2 Bund Parsley, smooth, cut

Preparation

- Put the carrot slices in a pot with a finger of water, bring to a boil, and cook over a low heat and with the lid closed for 7-8 minutes; drain off the water.

- Melt the herb butter; add the carrots and frozen peas, heat with stirring, salt, pepper and sugar, fold in the parsley.

45. Chicken and mushrooms with zucchini doodles soup

Ingredients (4 people)

- Thyme
- Salt pepper
- 4 tablespoons fresh cream
- 4 teaspoons flour
- 50cl of chicken broth
- 1/2 teaspoon of curry
- 600g of zucchini
- 600g of mushrooms
- 3 beautiful onions
- 600 g of chicken breast (turkey does as well)

Preparation

- Wash zucchini, peel mushrooms and onions, and mince all.
- Sauté the chicken in a casserole with a little oil, salt and add the curry, mix well. Remove from the pan, keep warm.
- In this same casserole saute the vegetables (zucchini, onions, mushrooms), after a few minutes add the chicken, add the broth, put the thyme, season and simmer covered.
- Mix the flour with the crème fraiche and at the end of the cooking, add this mixture to the chicken a little boil and serve hot.

46. Poached salmon with champagne

Preparation time: 10-15 mins

Makes 4 servings

Ingredients

- 4 salmon fillets (6 ounces each)
- 1 bottle (740 ml) of brut- type champagne, at room temperature

- ➤ 1 leek or garlic leek (leek), white part only finely cut
- ➤ 1 large shallot, finely chopped
- ➤ 1 lemon cut into wheels
- ➤ Star anise, only one star
- ➤ 6 branches of parsley
- ➤ 1 chile serrano cut in half (optional)
- ➤ 1 teaspoon salt
- ➤ ½ cup of cream (heavy cream)

To decorate

- ➤ 1 sprig of parsley

Preparation

1. Pour all ingredients except salmon and cream in a deep pan. Heat over high heat until the mixture boils. Lower to medium heat.

2. Carefully slide the salmon fillets into the champagne mixture. Cover the pan and cook for 4 minutes. Remove the salmon fillets. Do not discard the liquid from the pan.

3. Place ½ cup of the champagne broth in a small saucepan. Heat until it boils and adds the cream slowly. Lower to medium heat

and cook, constantly stirring, until thick. Try the sauce and add a pinch of salt, if you like.

4. If the salmon fillets have cooled, reheat the champagne broth and add the salmon fillets. Cook for one or two minutes, or till the salmon, is hot. Remove the fillets from the broth and serve on a plate.

5. Decorate each salmon fillet with a spoonful or two of the cream sauce and a leaf of parsley. Serve with salad or rice.

.

47. Custard with double chocolate
Preparation time: 10-15 mins

Makes 6 servings

Ingredients

- ➢ 2 cups whole milk
- ➢ 6 tablespoons of sugar
- ➢ 1/4 cup cocoa powder without sugar
- ➢ 2 tablespoons cornstarch
- ➢ 1 1/2 teaspoons cinnamon powder
- ➢ 1/8 teaspoon of salt

> ➢ 2 ounces of bitter chocolate
> ➢ 2 tablespoons toasted pumpkin seeds

Preparation

1. Heat the milk in a microwave in a 1-quart Pyrex cup until it almost boils, about 3 to 4 minutes. Meanwhile, beat the sugar, cocoa, cornstarch, cinnamon, and salt in a medium saucepan. At medium heat, add the milk and beat the mixture vigorously. Continue beating until the mixture reaches the consistency of the custard, about two minutes.

2. Remove from heat, add chocolate and beat more.

3. Serve hot or pour in an airtight container or in 6 custard cups covered with plastic to avoid a hard layer of cream. Sprinkle the pumpkin seeds on the custard before serving. It can be kept refrigerated for a maximum of 5 days.

48. Cucumber Salad, Cheese and Nuts

Preparation time: 15 minutes

Ingredients

- 100 g of cheese (at least 48% mg)
- 30 g of nuts
- 30 g of almonds
- 1 bag of salad of your choice
- ½ cup of mushrooms
- 2 tomatoes
- ¼ cucumber
- 4 c. corn
- 1 C. honey coffee
- 1 C. mustard
- 1 C. tablespoon of coconut oil

Preparation:

1. Cut the mushrooms into strips.
2. Heat the coconut oil inside a pan and fry the mushrooms briefly over high heat.
3. Slice tomatoes, cucumber, and the cheese into small cubes, chop the nuts finely.

4. In a salad bowl, put tomatoes, cucumber, cheese, nuts, almonds, mushrooms and corn. Stir well.
5. Prepare the vinaigrette by mixing honey, mustard and a little water.
6. Spread the salad on two plates and add the mixture of cheese, nuts, and vegetables.
7. Season with a little vinaigrette and your salad is ready.

49. Low Caramel Bread Recipe: Hemp and Psyllium Seeds

Preparation time: 70 minutes

Ingredients

- 5 eggs
- 150 g of fromage frais
- 5 c. tablespoon of olive oil
- 60 g ground flaxseed
- 60 g of wheat bran
- 40 g of nuts
- 1 C. sunflower seeds
- 1 C. squash seeds
- 1 C. hemp seeds

- 15 g of baking powder
- 30 g of protein powder
- 15 g of psyllium
- 4 c. tablespoons water

Preparation:

1. Preheat the oven to 160 ° C.
2. Mix the eggs, the fromage frais, and the olive oil until a homogeneous mixture.
3. Chop the nuts finely and add them to the mixture, then add the remaining ingredients.
4. Stir all and pour the dough into the mold.
5. Bake and then cook for 60 minutes.
6. Let the bread cool on a rack.

50. Eggplant Cutlets

For 4 person

Ingredients

4 eggplant

4 eggs

4 Plate of flour

Panko sign

Pinch of cumin

4 tablespoon parsley

800 gr tomatoes on a branch

4 tablespoon coarsely chopped almond

800 gr sweet mashed potatoes

Pepper and salt

Preparation

Heat the oven to 200 degrees. Cut the eggplant into small slices of 1 cm thick (6 pieces). Place them on a cutting board and sprinkle generously with salt. Let them lie for 20 minutes so that the moisture will come out. Then rinse and pat dry. Place the tomatoes with a branch in a baking dish and sprinkle with a little oil and pepper and salt and roast in the oven for 15 minutes. Beat the egg on a plate. Mix the flour with a pinch of pepper, salt, and cumin. Mix the parsley with the panko.

Get the eggplant slices through the flour first, then through the egg and then through the panko. Bake the aubergines in a frying pan with a little oil or margarine, about 5 minutes on each side, until its nicely golden brown. Heat the sweet mashed potatoes and put them on a plate, serve with the eggplant cutlets and the roasted tomatoes and garnish with some almond and a sprig of minced parsley.

Nutritional Facts

Calories 25   % Daily Value

Total Fat 0.2 g   0%

Saturated fat 0 g   0%

Polyunsaturated fat 0.1 g

Monounsaturated fat 0 g

Cholesterol 0 mg   0%

Sodium 2 mg   0%

Potassium 229 mg   6%

Total Carbohydrate 6 g   2%

Dietary fiber 3 g   12%

Sugar 3.5 g

Protein 1 g

51. Broccoli and lentils salad

Ingredients for 4 people

4 cup dried lentils,

2 onions,

4 bay leaves,

 4 broccolis divided into florets,

4 grated carrot,

Olive oil,

4 clove of garlic,

4 tablespoon of balsamic vinegar,

4 lemons,

 Salt, and pepper

Preparation

1. Our first step will be to cook the lentils. To do this, once washed, place them in the pressure cooker together with a liter of water, 1/4 onion, bay leaves, a spoonful of salt and a tablespoon of olive oil, cover and count 8 minutes later that the pot has reached its pressure point. If we do not have a pressure cooker, it will be enough to put them to boil inside

a covered pan for 30 minutes. Once cooked, drain and reserve.

2. While the lentils are cooking, we blanch the broccoli. Nothing is as simple as dipping the broccoli florets in boiling water for three minutes, then drain and immerse another three minutes in ice water. Next, we prepare vinaigrette with lemon juice, crushed garlic, balsamic vinegar, salt and pepper to taste.

3. Once the lentils and broccoli are cooked, and the carrot is grated, we proceed to assemble our salad. The secret of this one, in particular, is to give flavor to the lentils, reason why we will place them in a bowl, and we will bathe them with the vinaigrette, trying that they are covered completely; Let them rest like this for two minutes and then integrate the carrot and broccoli florets, stir and serve immediately.

Tasting

This fresh salad of broccoli and lentils is a recipe that has a very good balance both in texture and flavor.

The softness of the lentils contrasts with the crunchy texture of the carrot and broccoli, while the strong flavor of garlic, and then balsamic vinegar is softened by the acidity of the lemon and the sweetness of the carrot. To serve it, we will not need more than a glass of fresh water and enough time and attention to enjoy it.

Nutritional Facts

Calories: 5.8

% Daily Value

Total fat 0.0g 0.0%

Saturated Fat 0.0g 0.0%

Trans Fat 0.0g

Cholesterol 0.0mg 0.0%

Sodium 4.2mg 0.0%

Total Carbs 0.8g 0.3%

Dietary Fiber 0.7g 2.6%

Sugars 0.0g

Protein 0.3g

Vitamin A 1.6%

Vitamin C 10.0%

Calcium 1.0%

Iron 0.7%

52. Chickpeas with Spinach

Spinach with chickpeas is a typical dish of Spanish cuisine. It is a simple recipe but very tasty; also, this version is lighter.

Preparation: 5 mins

Cooking: 15 mins

Total: 20 minutes

Servings: 4

Ingredients

Extra virgin olive oil

1 head of garlic (12 teeth)

3 tablespoons of sweet paprika

6 cups of spinach (250 g)

1/2 cup of water (125 ml)

3 and 1/2 cups cooked chickpeas (650 g)

Salt (optional)

Preparation

1. In a pan add oil and when it is hot, add the chopped garlic. Cook over medium heat until golden brown.
2. Pour the paprika, stir and toss the chopped spinach. You can add plenty of oil so that the spinach is cooked or use 1/2 cup of water. Leave the spinach for about 5 minutes. You can also add salt, although I do not miss it.

3. Put the chickpeas, stir and if you want you can add a little more paprika or oil — Cook for about 5 more minutes.

Nutritional Facts

Total Fat: 5.8 g

Calories: 194.4

Dietary Fiber: 6.8 g

Saturated Fat: 0.5 g

Carbs: 10g

53. Thai Cucumber Salad

4 For person

Ingredients

4 large cucumber, cut in half and in thin half moons

12 tablespoons rice vinegar

4 tablespoons white sugar or honey

4 jalapeño pepper, seeded also finely chopped

2 orange bell pepper, in squares

4 tablespoons cilantro, chopped

2 cup peanuts

Salt and pepper to taste

2 pinch of chili flakes

Preparation

1. Mix rice vinegar and the sugar in a bowl until it has completely dissolved.
2. Cut the cucumber horizontally and then cut thin half-moons. (If you like, you can peel the cucumber).
3. Cut the jalapeño and the pepper.
4. Add the cucumber, jalapeño, bell pepper and the chili flakes in the bowl with the rice vinegar mixture and mix very well.
5. Season with salt and pepper to taste.
6. At the time of serving, add the cilantro and the chopped peanuts.

Nutritional Facts

Calories   55.6

Total Fat   0.2 g

Saturated Fat   0.0 g

Polyunsaturated Fat   0.0 g

Monounsaturated Fat   0.0 g

Cholesterol   0.0 mg

Sodium   267.8 mg

Potassium   190.4 mg

Total Carbohydrate   12.8 g

Dietary Fiber   1.2 g

Sugars   10.9 g

Protein   1.1 g

54. Grilled steak with red pepper

For 4 person

Ingredients

3 piece steak

3 roasted red peppers

For Sauce

1 tablespoon Worcestershire sauce

2 tablespoons honey

4 tablespoons balsamic vinegar

3 tablespoons of ketchup or hot sauce

1 teaspoon of dijon mustard

3 tablespoons olive oil

1 teaspoon of granulated sugar

Salt

Black pepper

Preparation

Mix the ingredients together for the sauce in a deep bowl. Place roasted peppers on each steak and wrap it in roll form. Cut the rolls in half and thread the bottle. Grill the steaks. When cooking both sides, apply with a brush from the sauce. Take your steaks to the serving plate.

Nutritional Information

Carbohydrates 10g 7.0%

Protein 48.0g 96%

55. Grilled Shrimp with Mint Sauce
For 4 people

Ingredients

 500 g shrimp

For Sauce

Half of fresh mint

1 ~ 2 shallots

3 cloves of garlic

2 tablespoons apple cider vinegar

1 tea glass of olive oil

1 teaspoon of sugar

2 teaspoons of salt

1 teaspoon of red paprika

Preparation

For the sauce, put all ingredients except olive oil into the blender and run the blender. Slowly add olive oil and have a thick consistency. Extract the shrimps and put them in a deep dish. Hover over the sauce and find all sides. Wrap the stretch film and leave in the refrigerator for at least 2-3 hours. Pass the prawns to the bottle. Cook on overheated grill. Serve hot.

Nutritional Information

Carbohydrates 10g 7.0%

Protein 40.0g 96%

56. Grilled sea bass with vegetables

For 4 person

Ingredients

4 perch

2 onion

4 cloves of garlic

2 potatoes

2 carrots

2 lemons

4 sprigs of rosemary

For Sauce

1 tea glass of olive oil

2 cloves of crushed garlic

1 teaspoon red ground pepper

1 teaspoon of red paprika

1 teaspoon black pepper

2 teaspoons of salt

Preparation

Clean the perch. Slice all vegetables to be very thin. You filled the fish with vegetables. Add the rosemary. Mix the ingredients for the sauce thoroughly with a fork. Tie the fish with the rope and take them to the barbecue. Brush with the help of the sauce you prepare and cook the fish duplex. Serve.

57. **Chicken Breast Grill with Soya**

58. Sauce

For 4 people

Ingredients

750 g chicken breast fillet

For Sauce:

2 tablespoons soy sauce

1 tablespoon honey

2 cloves of crushed garlic

1 teaspoon of grated fresh ginger

1 teaspoon of brown sugar

1 tea glass of olive oil

Salt

Black pepper

Preparation

Take the ingredients for the sauce in a deep bowl and mix. Chop the chicken breast into large pieces. Take the chicken meat into the bowl containing the sauce and mix. Stretch the film and let it rest in the refrigerator for 1 hour. Index of meats in bottles, cook on the grill. Serve hot.

Nutritional Information

Carbohydrates 20g 7.0%

Protein 48.0g 96%

59. Broccoli, Zucchini & Onions Soup: Super Healthy Recipe

Preparation time: 10-15 mins

Ingredients

- 150 g broccoli
- ½ courgette
- ½ red onion
- 1 C. tablespoon of coconut oil
- 400 ml of water
- 1 bouillon-cube with herbs

Preparation:

1. Cut the red onion and zucchini into small pieces.
2. Then cut the broccoli florets.
3. Heat the coconut oil inside a pan and fry the red onion for about 3 minutes. Then cook the zucchini for 5 minutes.
4. Add the broccoli florets, water, and bouillon cube. Simmer on low heat for 4 minutes.

5. Reduce everything to the blender until you get a creamy soup.
6. This broccoli, zucchini and onion soup can be served immediately or reheated later as you wish. Enjoy your meal!

60. Mint Strawberries with Green Asparagus

Ingredients

For 2-3 persons

- 1000 g asparagus (green)
- 500 g strawberries
- 2-3 fried eggs
- 250 g of ham (e.g., farmer's ham, cooked ham, etc.)
- some branches of fresh mint
- Salt pepper

Preparation

1. Wash the asparagus and then slice off the ends (woody taste).

Tip for women between 40 - 65:

There is a special program for interval fasting during menopause! The interval fast is combined with nutritional plans, so that the female body, despite the "menopause hormone conversion" goes back into the fat burning mode.

2. Wash the strawberries, cut the stalk and halve or quarter as desired. Slice the mint and then mix it with the strawberries.
3. Use a large pot of salted water to the boil, add the asparagus, bring to a boil and cook over medium heat for 5-7 minutes.
4. Heat a pan with butter and fry the fried eggs over medium heat and lid.
5. Hams are enough.

61. Hot chocolate with coconut

Makes 2 servings

Do not confuse the coconut drink with milk or canned coconut cream. The coconut drink is almost always found in the non-dairy milk section.

Ingredients

2 cups of coconut drink (like Coconut Dream)

2 ounces of bitter chocolate

1 pinch of salt

1 teaspoon vanilla extract

Preparation

Mix the coconut drink, chocolate, and salt and simmer the mixture in a medium saucepan, whisking until the chocolate melts. Remove from heat, add vanilla and serve.

62. Milk recipe

Preparation time: 30 min

Ingredients

- 1 l of pasteurized whole milk
- 100 ml of bought thick milk

Preparation

Put the milk in a bowl or a wide jug. Stir in the used milk with the whisk and let the milk stand at room temperature for approx. 20 hours and let it thicken. Then it can be spooned or drunk or enriched with fruit without any further ingredients.

63. Plaice rolls with celeriac and rucola puree

Preparation: 40 min

Calories: 272 kcal

Rucola is rich in folic acid and other B vitamins. Through its bitter substances, the herb stimulates the digestion and also acts dehydrating. The tender fish contains a lot of high-quality protein; the tomatoes score with cell-protecting lycopene.

Ingredients

- For four portions
- One piece celeriac (400 g)
- salt
- 5 tbsps.
- lemon juice
- 125 g arugula
- 3 tbsps. olive oil
- 50 ml of vegetable stock
- 2 tbsps. light sesame seeds (30 g)
- 100 g yellow cocktail tomatoes
- 50 ml milk (3.5% fat)
- Pepper
- Two plaice fillets (approx. 150 g each)

Preparation

- Clean the celeriac, peel, cut into pieces and cook in salted water with one tablespoon of lemon juice for 10-15 minutes over medium heat.

- Meanwhile, clean the rocket, wash and spin dry, removing coarse stems; Place half of the rocket leaves in a high mixing bowl and set the rest aside. Add one tablespoon of oil and vegetable broth to the rocket in the mixing bowl and puree everything with a hand blender.

- Roast sesame seeds in a hot pan with no fat on low heat. Wash tomatoes and halve.

- Drain the celery and let it evaporate. Then crush in a saucepan with milk and mix in 1 tbsp. oil and rucola puree. Season the puree with salt, pepper and one tablespoon of lemon juice.

- Rinse plaice fillets, dab dry, halve each lengthwise and lightly salt and pepper. Spread each fish fillet strip with 1/4 of the celery and rocket puree, roll up loosely and fix with roulade skewers or wooden skewers. Place fish rolls next to each other in a small baking dish, place the tomatoes and then cook in a pre-heated oven at 180 ° C (circulating air 160 ° C, gas: stage 2-3) for 15-20 minutes.

- In the meantime arrange the put aside rucola on plates. Make a dressing with remaining lemon juice, salt, pepper and remaining oil and drizzle with rocketroot leaves. Remove roulades from the oven, arrange with the tomatoes on the rocket salad and sprinkle with sesame seeds.

64. Mushroom and vegetable pan with almonds

Preparation: 30 min

Calories: 203 kcal

The colorful mixture of vegetables and mushrooms contains plenty of fiber, which ensures long-lasting satiety. Peppers also provide plenty of immunes boosting vitamin C; the carrots score with beta carotene, a precursor of vitamin A. The fat-soluble vitamin is essential for healthy eyes, among other things.

Ingredients

For four portions

- One big onion
- Two garlic cloves
- Three tomatoes
- One red pepper
- Two parsley
- Two carrots

- Salt
- 2 tbsps. almonds (40 g)
- 400 g mixed mushrooms
- 1 tbsp. butter (15 g)
- Pepper
- 1 splash
- Lemon juice
- ½ tbsp.
- Curry powder
- 2 tbsps.
- Sour cream (40 g)

Preparation

- Peel onion and garlic and chop finely. Wash the tomatoes and slice into small cubes. Wash the pepper, clean and cut into thin strips.

- Peel parsley roots and carrots, cut into thin sticks and blanch in boiling salted water for 2 minutes. Drain, quench and drain.

- Meanwhile roast almonds in a pan over medium heat without fat until they smell.

- Clean and slice mushrooms. Heat the butter in a pan. Fry the onion and garlic over at medium heat until glassy. Add the pepper and simmer for 3 minutes.

- Add mushrooms and simmer for 3-4 minutes over medium heat until they are ready. Add tomatoes, carrots and parsley roots and simmer for another 2 minutes. Season with salt, pepper, one dash of lemon juice and curry powder.

- Add mushrooms and simmer for 3-4 minutes over medium heat until they are ready. Add tomatoes, carrots and parsley roots and simmer for another 2 minutes. Season with salt, pepper, one dash of lemon juice and curry powder.

- Stir in sour cream and sprinkle with almonds.

65. Vegetable Burgers

Cooking time: 30 to 60 min

Ingredients

- 250g vegetables (carrots, zucchini, leeks, peas, corn, carob,)

- 70 g of oatmeal (roughly chopped)

- 20 g of butter

- 125 ml of milk

- 1-piece egg

- 100 g crumbs (of debarked white bread)

- Salt

- Pepper

- Marjoram

- 1 tbsp. parsley (freshly chopped)

- Crumbs (to roll)

- Oil (or clarified butter for frying)

Preparation:

- Depending on the consistency, grate the vegetables roughly or cut them into small pieces and possibly boil them up. Sweat the oats in butter, pour milk on them and let them boil down. Let cool down. Then mix with vegetables and the egg and tie with the crumbs, season with spicy salt, pepper, marjoram, and parsley.

- From the mass patties (small patties) form, dip one side in breadcrumbs and fry in air fryer.

- Suggested side: Tomato or warm or cold herb sauce, the patties can also be served as a side dish to vegetable dishes with sauce.

Nutritional Information:

- Calories 177

- Total Fat 6 g 9%

- Saturated fat 1.4 g 7%

- Polyunsaturated fat 2 g

- Monounsaturated fat 1.8 g

- Cholesterol 5 mg

- Sodium 569 mg

- Potassium 333 mg

- Total Carbohydrate 14 g

- Dietary fiber 4.9 g

- Sugar 1.1 g

- Protein 16 g

- Vitamin A 0%

- Vitamin C 7%

- Calcium 13%

- Iron 13%

- Vitamin D 0%

- Vitamin B-6 15%

66. Meatball with parsley carrots

Ingredients for four servings

• Three onions

• 500 g of beefsteak minced meat

• 4 tbsps. Of breadcrumbs

• 2 tsp. mustard

• Salt

• Pepper

• 4 Tbsps. oil

• 800 g of carrots

• 400 grams of romaine lettuce

• One bunch of parsley

Preparation

• Dice the onions

• Hack, breadcrumbs, half onion and mustard knead.

• Season with salt and pepper

• Make four meatballs. Heat 2 tablespoons of oil, fry the 10 minutes.

• Meanwhile, cut carrots into slices. Stew onions and carrots in 2 tablespoons of oil, season. Pour 400 ml of water; simmer until the liquid evaporates. Cut salad and parsley into strips. Mix and taste it.

Per serving about 350 kcal

67. Salmon fillet with mustard crust

Ingredients for four servings

• Two red peppers

• 700 g of potatoes

• 10 g herb butter

• 120 ml broth

• Two stems of rosemary

- 100 g of frozen peas

- Four pieces (a ca. 150 g)

- Salmon fillet

- Salt

- Pepper

- 1 tbsp. oil

- five tablespoons coarse mustard

- 3 tbsps breadcrumbs

Preparation

- Cut the peppers into strips. Peel potatoes, slice. Cover potatoes, herb butter, broth and rosemary needles and simmer for about 10 minutes. Add peas and pepper after approx. 7 minutes.

- Season salmon with salt and pepper.

Heat oil, sear salmon on both sides, put on a baking tray. Mix mustard and breadcrumbs spread the fish over it and gratin ate under the hot grill for 3 to 4 minutes. Season vegetables, serve with fish.

Per serving about 500 kcal

68. Soup cream of palm heart

Whether winter or summer, slimming soups are always looked light, healthy and easily digestible meal.

They offer another benefit: they can be used during a diet to lose weight, with high nutrients and few calories that bring about satiety of the body without gaining weight.

Ingredients

- 250 grams of Pupunha palm
- 3 cups chicken broth tea
- 1 cup skim milk
- 1 tbsp light margarine
- One grated onion
- One garlic clove, minced
- Two tablespoons wheat flour
- Small salt

Preparation

- The onion and garlic should be sautéed in light margarine. Next, add the palm heart and fry a bit more to absorb the taste of the spice.
- It takes 2 to 3 minutes.
- Dissolve the wheat flour in the chicken broth. Add the sautéed palm hearts. Let cook for about 10 minutes;
- When it is lukewarm, it is time to liquefy all this by adding the milk. Back to the fire for another 5 or 6 minutes. It's time to taste the salt. Serve immediately.

Yield: 6 servings (1 medium Conch)

Calories per serving: about 62 calories

69. Vegetables and vegetables slimming soup

Ingredients

- 250 ml of water;
- One medium carrot;
- One small potato;
- One large sheet of cabbage butter
- One large cabbage leaf
- Two teaspoons of olive oil
- Small salt.

Preparation

Boil all ingredients in the water. Then liquidate everything.

Yield: 1 part

Calories per serving: 58 calories.

70. Chicken soup with ginger

Ingredients

- Two cooked chicken steaks and minced
- Four tablespoons of cooked and chopped carrots
- 3 cups chicken roast water
- One tablespoon of oil
- One small piece of ginger (not much larger than a hazelnut), unless you love the spicy taste of this root
- One grated onion
- One garlic clove, minced
- One tablespoon cornstarch
- Small salt

Preparation

First, the onion and garlic should be sautéed in the oil. Incidentally, the carrot should be cooked in the blender with two cups of chicken stock. Next, this cream should be added to the onion and garlic porridge. At this point, the ginger included the recipe, and everything should cook for a few minutes.

In the meantime, the cornstarch should be dissolved to the other broth from the remaining chicken jerk. At this moment, it is boiled and continuously stirred until it thickens. At the last minute, incorporate the chicken, taste the salt and serve immediately.

Yield: 4 servings

Calories per serving: about 150 calories

71. Zucchini with yogurt dip

Preparation: 25 min

Calories: 193 kcal

Zucchini contains around 90% water as well as hematopoietic iron and nerve-strengthening magnesium. Yogurt, with its lactic acid bacteria, soothes the intestines and promotes digestion.

Ingredients

- For four portions
- Three zucchini (700 g)
- 2 tbsps. olive oil
- ½ lemon (juice)
- salt
- pepper
- One handful mint (5 g)
- 1 tsp. sambal oelek
- 500 g yogurt (1.5% fat)
- One pomegranate (250 g)

Preparation

- Clean, wash and slice the zucchini. Mix the zucchini slices with oil and lemon juice and season with salt and pepper.

- Heat a grill pan. Fry the zucchini in slices on both sides for 2-3 minutes over medium heat.

- Wash mint, shake dry, peel off leaves, put aside some for garnish. Chop the rest for the dip and stir in the yogurt with Sambal oelek, then season with one pinch of salt and pepper.

- Halve the pomegranate and then remove the seeds from the fruit. Arrange the zucchini slices on plates and drizzle with the yogurt dip. Spread the pomegranate seeds over them and garnish with mint leaves.

72. Monkfish and spinach parcels

Preparation: 45 min

Calories: 351 kcal

The sea fish provides plenty of iodine and protein. Both ensure a smooth flow of metabolism. The spicy-tasting leek is very rich in zinc and thus has a wound-healing an immune-boosting effect.

Ingredients

- For four portions
- 50 g spinach
- salt
- 2 bars leek
- Two big carrots (300 g)
- 600 g monkfish
- One organic lemon
- 300 g seelachsfilet
- 100 ml of soy cream
- 150 g cottage cheese (0.3% fat)
- Pepper
- 100 ml fish stock (glass)
- 250 g yellow or red cherry tomatoes
- 1 tbsp. olive oil
- Four red sorrel orchard leaves at will
- ¼ bunch chives (5 g)

Preparation

- Clean, wash and drizzle the spinach in boiling salted water and let it collapse in 1-2 minutes. Remove spinach, chill cold, squeeze well, chop and chill.

- Clean the leeks cut in length and wash. Separate the leaves from each other and add to the boiling salted water for 2 minutes. Then remove cold quench and dab dry.

- Clean and peel the carrots, cut lengthways into thin strips and add to the boiling salted water for 3 minutes until soft. Remove, chill off cold and dab carrot strips dry.

- Wash monkfish fillet and pat dry. Lay the bottom of an ovenproof mold slightly overlapping with the leek and carrot strips. Place the monkfish filet in the middle of it.

- Rinse the lemon hot, rub dry, rub the skin and squeeze juice. Cut the salmon filet into small pieces and puree with soy cream, cottage cheese and spinach to a fine mass. Season the mixture with salt, pepper, lemon peel, and juice, spread on the fillet and beat the vegetable strips over the fish from both sides.

- Add fish stock and cook the monkfish fillet in a preheated oven at 180 ° C (160 ° C convection, gas: stage 2-3) for about 30 minutes.

- In the meantime wash and halve cherry tomatoes. In a frying pan, fry the tomatoes in it for about 5 minutes over medium heat.

- Wash lettuce leaves and chives and shake dry. Cut monkfish fillet in leek and carrot clove into four pieces and arrange with tomatoes, lettuce leaves, and chives.

73. Romaine lettuce with radishes and avocado yogurt sauce

Preparation: 35 min

Calories: 177 kcal

Due to its lactic acid bacteria, yogurt has a beneficial effect on the intestine and promotes digestion. Also, the dairy product is rich in calcium and a good source of protein. With the high-fat avocado, good fats, lots of potassium and vitamin E are in the salad.

Ingredients

For four portions

- Two green peppers
- 1 tbsp. white wine vinegar
- 1 tbsp. olive oil
- Four eggs
- ½ clove of garlic
- One lime
- ¼ ripe avocado (50 g)
- 200 g yogurt (0.3% fat)
- some splash of Worcester sauce
- salt

- pepper
- One head romaine lettuce (300 g)
- One red onion
- One bunch radish
- ½ bunch coriander (10 g)
- 2 tsps. pickled green pepper (glass, 10 g)

Preparation

- Slice the peppers into half, corer them, wash them and grill with the skin side up in the preheated oven with the grill function until the paprika skin is black. Then allow cooling slightly. Peel off the skin, finely chop the pepper and marinate with vinegar and olive oil for about 15 minutes.

- Meanwhile, boil eggs in 8-10 minutes. Then put off, peel and cut into slices.

- In the meantime peel garlic for the sauce and finely chop. Halve the lime and squeeze juice. Remove the core of the avocado and lift the flesh out of the shell. Puree garlic, lime juice, avocado, yogurt and Worcester sauce with a hand blender. Season the sauce with salt and pepper.

- Clean the lettuce, wash, cut into small pieces and spin dry. Peel the onion, halve and cut into strips. Clean radishes, wash and slice them. Wash cilantro, shake dry and peel off leaves.

- Mix salad with diced peppers and serve on plates. Spread onions, eggs and radishes on top. Drizzle with the sauce spread the green pepper and garnish with coriander leaves.

74. Chicken breast with avocado and cauliflower mash

Chicken Breast with Avocado and Cauliflower Stomp, tender poultry with an aromatic side dish just delicious and made fast!

Preparation: 25 min

Calories: 294 kcal

Although the avocado is high in calories and high in fat, it is excellent for fasting because it has plenty of vitamin E, potassium and good fats. The tender chicken provides plenty of protein; the cheese contains a lot of bone-strengthening calcium.

Ingredients

- For four portions
- ½ cauliflower (600 g)
- salt
- One onion
- 50 g sun-dried tomatoes

- 2 tbsps. rapeseed oil
- pepper
- Four chicken breast fillets (à 125 g)
- Three tbsps. lemon juice
- 80 ml milk (3.5% fat)
- 80 ml of vegetable stock
- ½ ripe avocado
- 80 g feta (9% fat)
- chives tip

Preparation

- Clean and wash the cauliflower, divide into florets and cook gently in a little salted water over medium heat for 8-10 minutes. Then drain.

- Meanwhile, peel and dice the onion. Slice tomatoes inside small pieces, heat little oil into a pan, sauté onions and tomatoes for 2 minutes over medium heat. Salt, pepper, and remove from the pan.

- Rinse chicken breast fillets, pat dry, salt and pepper, heat remaining oil in the pan. Fry the meat on both sides for 5-8 minutes over medium heat. Sprinkle with lemon juice and remove the pan from the heat; Cover the meat and let it spread.

- Warm milk with broth, remove the core from the avocado and lift the pulp out of the shell. Cauliflower and avocado meat in a bowl, mash with a fork, mix in the warm milk stock and season with salt and pepper.

- Spread the stomping on plates for serving and put the chicken breast on top. Sprinkle onion-tomato mixture, crumble feta and spread over it. Garnish with chives and sprinkle with pepper as you like.

75. Pepper with cottage cheese

Preparation: 15 minutes

Calories: 140 kcal

The granular cream cheese, also called cottage cheese, is especially popular with athletes. The crunchy peppers provide us with plenty of vitamin C, which is of great importance for an intact immune system.

Ingredients

For four portions

- One red onion (50 g)
- ½ small lemon (juice)
- 150 g grainy cream cheese (0.8% fat)
- 150 g low-fat quark
- ½ tl mild curry powder
- Salt
- One pinch cayenne pepper
- Two small yellow peppers (à ca. 150 g)
- Two little red pepper (à ca. 150 g)

- Four stems dill
- One heaped el pine nuts (20 g)

Preparation

- Peel the onions and slice them. Stir lemon juice with cream cheese, curd cheese and 3-4 tablespoons of water in a bowl until smooth. Add the onion, season with curry, salt, and cayenne pepper.

- Cut peppers in half, core and wash. Wash dill, shake dry and chop. Roast pine nuts without fat in a pan over medium heat.

- Fill paprika halves with the cottage cheese mixture and serve them sprinkled with dill and pine nuts.

76. Rocket salad with mango, avocado and cherry tomatoes

Preparation: 15 minutes

Calories: 306 kcal

Although avocados contain a lot of fat, because in addition to plenty of vitamin E score the green fruits with healthy polyunsaturated fatty acids, Mango has its yellow color due to the plant pigment beta carotene, which is a precursor of vitamin A, which is vital for healthy eyes. The cell-protecting lycopene from tomatoes completes the essential substance package.

Ingredients

For four portions

- 1 tbsp. lime juice
- 2 tbsps. white balsamic vinegar
- 2 tbsps. rapeseed oil
- 2 tbsps. olive oil
- 1 tsp. honey

- 1 tsp. medium hot mustard
- Salt
- Pepper
- Three handful rocket (120 g)
- 200 g cherry tomatoes
- One ripe mango
- Two avocados

Preparation

- For the vinaigrette, whip lime juice with vinegar and both oils. Whisk in honey and mustard and then season with salt and pepper.

- Wash the rocket and spin dry. Wash tomatoes and halve. Peel the mango, slice the pulp from the core and dice it. Halve the avocados, core them, remove the pulp from the skin and dice them as well. Add all the salad ingredients inside a bowl with the vinaigrette and spread on four plates.

77. Simple fruit salad

Cooking time: 15 to 30 min

Ingredients

Portions: 1

- One pear

- One apple

- One piece of banana

- Sesame

- Cinnamon

Preparation

For the fruit salad, first cut all fruits into small pieces and mix in a bowl. Sprinkle cinnamon and sesame on top and place in the air fryer for 30 sec to steam; then a delicious snack is ready in between.

Tip

With honey, the fruit salad tastes great too!

Nutritional Information:

- Calories   97
- 1%Total Fat   0.5g grams
- 0% Saturated   Fat 0.1g grams
- Trans Fat   0g grams
- Polyunsaturated Fat   0.2g grams
- Monounsaturated Fat   0.1g grams
- 0%Cholesterol   0mg milligrams
- 8%Total Carbohydrates   24g grams
- 13% Dietary Fiber   3.3g grams
- Sugars   16g grams
- Protein   1.4g grams
- 1.9% Vitamin A
- 120% Vitamin C
- 2% Calcium
- 2.9% Iron

78. Potato Gratin from the Hot Air Fryer

Cooking time: 15 to 30 min

Ingredients

Servings: 4

- 400 g potatoes (slightly floury, peeled)

- 50 ml of milk

- 50 ml whipping cream

- Pepper (freshly ground)

- Nutmeg

- 40 g Gruyere cheese (or middle-aged cheese, grated)

Preparation:

- For the potato gratin, cut the potatoes into thin slices.

- Mix the milk in a bowl with whipped cream and season with salt, pepper, and nutmeg. Turn the sliced potatoes in the milk mixture.

• Put the slices of potatoes in a slightly oiled quiche (15 cm diameter) and pour the rest of the topping from the bowl over the potatoes. Distribute the cheese evenly over the potatoes.

• Place the quiche dish in the cooking basket and push the basket into the air fryer. Set the timer to 15-20 minutes and bake the potato gratin at 200°C, until it is beautifully browned and cooked.

Preparation: time: 10 minutes + 15 minutes in the hot air fryer.

Nutritional Information:

• Calories 323

• 29% Total Fat 18.6g

• 58% Saturated Fat 11.6g

• 19% Cholesterol 56mg

• 46% Sodium 1061mg

- 9% Total Carbohydrate 27.6g

- 16% Dietary Fiber 4.4g

- Protein 12.4g

- 13% Vitamin A 647 IU

- 40% Vitamin C 24mg

- 29% Calcium 292mg

- 9% Iron 1.6mg

79. Avocado cold soup with walnuts

- Ingredient
- 200 grams of chopped avocado
- 200 ml of ice-cold coconut water
- Half lemon juice
- One tablespoon of chopped walnuts
- Extra virgin olive oil.

Preparation

Avocado, coconut water, and lemon all blend with the blender. Then spread the walnuts and pour a filet extra virgin olive oil.

Yield: 2 servings

Calories per serving: about 223 calories

80. Cold soup of zucchini with tomato

Ingredients

- 1 cup of chopped tomatoes (with or without seeds, according to taste, although the seeds are a source of insoluble fiber);
- One raw zucchini in thin slices (the finer, the more interesting the result);
- One teaspoon of capers
- One fillet of extra virgin olive oil;
- Small salt

Preparation

Blend the tomato in the blender with a cup of water. Next, add olive oil and salt. Add zucchini bananas and capers to this mixture. Serve with ice cubes.

Yield: 2 servings

Calories per serving: about 36 calories

81. Fish in sesame crust with carrot and avocado salad

Preparation: 30 min

Calories: 587 kcal

The tender fish contains plenty of protein, which is needed for muscle building. Avocados, olive and sesame oil score with vitamin E and healthy polyunsaturated fatty acids.

Ingredients

- For four portions
- Two carrots
- 100 g arugula
- Two avocados
- 2 tbsps.
- balsamic vinegar
- 1 tbsp.
- lemon juice
- 1 tbsp.
- olive oil
- salt
- pepper
- 600 g white fish fillet (e.g., zander)
- 3 tbsps. whole wheat flour (45 g)

- 80 g sesame
- Two eggs
- 4 tbsps.
- sesame oil
- ½ bunches
- Basil (10 g)

Preparation

- Peel carrots and finely grate. Wash the rocket and spin dry. Halve the avocados, remove seeds, peel and cut into bite-sized pieces. Mix carrot, rocket and avocado slices in a bowl with vinegar, lemon juice and olive oil and season of giving a taste with salt and pepper. Distribute on four plates.

- Rinse fish with cold water, pat dry and then cut into 12 equal pieces. Fill flour and sesame into 2 deep plates, whisk eggs in a deep dish. Salt and pepper the fish. Then turn in the flour, pull through the eggs and bread with sesame seeds. Heat the oil with a non-stick pan and then fry the fish pieces in a medium heat from each side until golden brown for 2-3 minutes.

- Wash basil, shake dry and peel off leaves. Drain the fish pieces briefly on paper towels, then place on the salad and sprinkle with basil.

82. Thai steak salad with herbs and onions

Preparation: 25 min

Coriander has a detoxifying effect and supports the removal of toxins. Ginger and chili make with their pungent materials for proper circulation and stimulate fat burning.

Ingredients

For four portion

- One flank or rump steak (600 g)
- Salt

- 1 tbsp. peanut oil
- Two red onions
- 1 piece
- Ginger (20 g)
- One red chili pepper
- One cucumber
- 3 handful
- Asian herbs (30 g)
- 1 tbsp. rice vinegar
- 3 tbsps. lime juice
- 2 tbsps.
- Fish sauce
- 1 tsp. honey
- Paprika
- Chili powder
- Pepper

Preparation

- Rinse meat, pat dry and salt. Heat the oil and then fry the steak on both sides for 6-8 minutes over high heat. Remove meat from the frying pan and let it rest.

- Meanwhile, peel onions and ginger. Halve onions and cut into strips.

Chop ginger. Cut chili pepper into half lengthwise remove seeds, wash and cut into fine rings. Clean the cucumber, wash, quarter it and slice it. Wash herbs, shake dry and peel off leaves.

- Add ginger with vinegar, lime juice, fish sauce, honey and 2-3 tablespoons water to a dressing, season with paprika, chili powder, salt, including pepper.

- Slice the meat and arrange with herbs, chili rings, cucumber and onions on a plate and drizzle with the dressing.

Calories: 390 kcal

83. Cucumber rolls on cauliflower salad

Preparation: 35 min

Calories: 246 kcal

This low-carb dish scores with low carbohydrates and many vitamins and minerals. Avocado and olive oil also contain plenty of healthy unsaturated fatty acids.

Ingredients

For four portions

- Two small cucumbers (600 g)
- One carrot
- ½ orange pepper
- One pole celery
- One avocado
- 2 tbsps.
- Sprouts
- Salt
- Pepper
- One cauliflower
- 50 g raisins
- 3 tbsps.
- Olive oil
- 3 tbsps. lemon juice
- 1 msp. Ground cumin
- One pinch cinnamon

- Chili flakes
- 4 stems parsley

Preparation

- Clean cucumbers, wash them and slice or slice lengthwise into skinny slices; Cut the slices of cucumber into narrow, long strips.

- Peel carrot. Halve, corer and wash the pepper. Clean and wipe the celery stick. Cut everything into thin finger-length strips.

- Halve the avocado, remove the core, remove the pulp from the skin and cut into small slices. Wash and rinse sprouts thoroughly. Bundle some vegetable strips and wrap with a few shots in 1 slice of cucumber, season with salt and pepper. Keep cold until serving.

- Clean cauliflower, wash and divide into small florets. Prepare the cauliflower in boiling salted water for about 5 minutes. Then drain, quench and let cool. Finely chop cauliflower, mix with raisins and oil. Season the cabbage with lemon juice, salt, pepper, cumin, cinnamon, and chili flakes.

- Wash parsley, shake dry and chop leaves. Spread cauliflower on a plate. Add 2-3 cucumber rolls and parsley.

84. Chili beef pan

Preparation: 15 minutes

Finished in 55 min

Calories: 450 kcal

Beef contains a lot of protein as well as large amounts of iron. The trace element it needs among other things for blood formation. Peppers score with immune-boosting vitamin C; the tomatoes deliver cell-protecting lycopene.

Ingredients

For 4 portions

- 6 pointed pepper (yellow and red)
- 1 red chili pepper
- 1 onion
- 1 clove of garlic
- 200 g cherry tomatoes
- 800 g lean beef (e.g. rump steak)
- 3 tbsps. olive oil
- 1 tbsp. tomato paste (20 g)
- 2 tbsps.
- Noble sweet paprika powder
- 750 ml of meat soup
- Salt
- Pepper
- Ground Coriander
- Ground caraway
- ½ bunch parsley (10 g)

Preparation

- Wash peppers, clean and cut into strips. Wash, clean and finely chop the chili pepper. Peel onion and garlic. Finely chop the onion and finely chop garlic. Wash, clean and halve tomatoes.

- Dab meat dries with kitchen paper and cuts into bite-sized strips. Then heat a little oil inside a pan and sauté the meat in portions over high heat for 2-3 minutes. Then take it out of the pan.

- Pure one tbsp. of oil to the pan, and sauté the chili, onion, and then add garlic over medium heat. Add the tomato puree and paprika powder and sauté for 1 minute. Pour broth, add meat, paprika and tomatoes and season with salt, pepper, coriander, and cumin. Simmer over minimum heat for about 35 minutes. Stir in between and add some broth if necessary.

- Meanwhile, wash parsley, shake dry and chop. Season the pepper-beef pan with salt and pepper, sprinkle with parsley and serve immediately.

85. Crispy Chicken Thighs with Bacon

Ingredient

- Four chicken drumsticks (s)
- Eight slices/ s Bacon, about 100 g
- Herbs, Mediterranean (rosemary, thyme, oregano, lavender)
- sea salt
- 1 tbsp. olive oil

Cooking time: approx. 50 min

Calorie: about 300 kcal

Preparation

- Preheat oven at 180 ° C (160 ° C convection). Wash the chicken thighs and pat dry.
- Heat the olive oil in the frying pan (if oven suitable) and fry the legs from all sides. Remove from the pan, season well all around (freshly chopped Mediterranean herbs or a high-quality dry mix) and salt. Then wrap with two slices of bacon, if necessary fix with wooden toothpicks, roast again in the still hot pan from above and below. Be careful when turning.
- Put the pan inside the oven for 30 minutes and add a touch of olive oil if necessary. If there is no pan suitable for cooking, place the legs on the oven rack and push a sheet of baking paper under it as a safety catch, after half the time turn the thighs. Serve hot!

It fits a light raw food salad.

Tip:

Do not use a casserole dish (used in the photo only for decorative purposes). In this, the thighs swim too much in their juice and are therefore not crispy.

Nutritional Information per Piece
- 300 kcal
- 16 g fat (of which 6 g total fat)
- KH 600 mg
- Protein 40 g

86. Cucumber salad

Preparation time: 10 minutes

Total time: 10 minutes

Ingredients

1 small red onion, sliced into thin slices

2 cucumbers, peeled or not (depending on the variety of cucumber and its taste), and cut into thin slices

Juice of 2-3 medium lemons

2 tablespoons chopped coriander finely (you can also use parsley)

2 tablespoons of olive oil

Salt to taste

Preparation

4. Put the onion slices in a dish and sprinkle with half a tablespoon of salt. Rub the onions with the salt and then cover them with water for a few minutes. Then sift and rinse the

onions well. This helps to remove the bitter and strong flavor of the onions.

5. Mix cucumber slices, washed onion, lemon juice, chopped coriander, and olive oil.3Mix well and then adjust the salt to taste.

6. The salad can be served immediately, or it can be left to rest for at least 30 minutes before serving.

Nutrition

Net carbohydrates: 3% (6 g)

Fiber: 5 g

Fat: 79% (67 g)

Protein: 18% (35 g)

kcal: 774

87. Corn salad, potatoes, and broccoli

Yield: For 2

Ingredients

1 cups corn kernels or fresh corn, almost 4 ears of corn, steamed or boiled

2 cups cooked potatoes, diced, about 3 medium potatoes

2 cups of broccoli flowers, lightly steamed or boiled

½ cup finely chopped red onion

2 tablespoons mayonnaise (you can also use plain yogurt)

1 garlic cloves, crushed

1 tablespoons coriander or finely chopped cilantro

1 tablespoons of lemon juice

½ teaspoon of wasabi pasta (or you can use horseradish / spicy mustard), fit to taste

Salt and pepper to taste

Preparation

- To prepare the dressing, combine the mayonnaise, crushed garlic, chopped coriander, lemon juice, wasabi paste, salt, and pepper inside a small bowl and then mix well.
- In a large salad bowl, add corn or fresh corn, potatoes, broccoli, and chopped onion.
- Add mayonnaise dressing with wasabi, mix well and serve immediately or refrigerate until meal time.

Nutrition

Energy   1480kj

Carbohydrates: 4% (7 g)

Fiber: 3 g

Fat: 77% (57 g)

Protein: 19% (32 g)

kcal: 674

88. Italian keto meatballs with mozzarella cheese

Tomato sauce, rich and comforting. Mozzarella, fresh and creamy. Meatballs, with the right touch of onion and oregano. It's like eating spaghetti, but without carbohydrates. Enjoy every bite, ketolicious!

Ingredients

450 g ground beef

50 g grated Parmesan cheese

1 egg

½ tbsp. dried basil

½ tsp. ground onion

1 tsp. garlic powder

1 tsp. Salt

½ tsp. ground black pepper

3 tbsps. olive oil

400 g canned whole tomatoes

2 tbsps. fresh parsley, finely chopped

200 g fresh spinach

50 g butter

150 g (325 ml) fresh mozzarella cheese

Salt and pepper

Preparation

Place the ground beef, Parmesan cheese, eggs, salt and spices in a bowl and mix well. Assemble the meatballs with the mixture, approximately 30 grams (1 ounce) each. It is easier if you have your hands moist while you make the meatballs.

Heat the olive oil in a large pan and sauté the meatballs until golden brown on all sides.

Reduce heat and add canned tomatoes. Then it let simmer for 15 minutes, stirring every couple of minutes. Salpimentar to taste. Add the parsley and stir. You can prepare the dish here to freeze it.

Melt the butter in another pan and fry the spinach for 1-2 minutes, stirring continuously. Salpimentar to taste. Add spinach to meatballs. Cover with fresh mozzarella cheese, cut into bite-sized pieces. Serve and enjoy.

Nutrition

Low carb ketogenic

Per portion

Net carbohydrates: 3% (5 g)

Fiber: 3 g

Fat: 72% (50 g)

Protein: 25% (39 g)

kcal: 628

89. Crispy Cheese Omelette

Once you've tried this omelette, there will be no going back. Its irresistible crust and sumptuous filling will make it your favorite omelette. It is ideal for a good breakfast, but it is also a great option for a quick keto dinner.

Ingredients

Omelette

2 eggs

2 tbsps. whipping cream

1 tbsps. butter or coconut oil

Salt and ground black pepper

75 g grated or sliced cheese, cured

Filling

2 sliced mushrooms

2 sliced cherry tomatoes

2 tbsp (30 g) cream cheese

15 g spinach sprouts

30 g turkey cold cuts

1 tsp. Dried oregano

Preparation

Inside a bowl beat the eggs, cream, salt and pepper.

Heat a tablespoon of butter in a nonstick skillet. Spread the cheese evenly in the pan to cover the entire bottom. Fry over medium heat until bubbly.

Carefully incorporate the egg mixture over the cheese and reduce heat. Cook a few minutes without stirring.

Fill half with mushrooms, tomatoes, spinach, cream cheese, turkey and oregano. Fry a few more minutes.

When the egg mixture begins to set (it can still be quite loose on top, but not too much), turn the empty half over half with the ingredients, forming a half moon. Fry a few more minutes and enjoy!

Nutrition

Low carb ketogenic

Per portion

Net carbohydrates: 4% (8 g)

Fiber: 2 g

Fat: 75% (66 g)

Protein: 21% (41 g)

kcal: 791

90. Steamed Cod

Preparation: 30 min

Calories: 226 kcal

The high-quality protein in the cod stimulates the metabolism and serves as a building material for cells, muscles, enzymes, and hormones. Valuable proteins also prevent cravings and muscle breakdown.

Ingredients

- For four portions
- Four cod fillets (à 150 g)
- 4 tbsps. lemon juice
- 2 bars leek
- 3 tbsps. rapeseed oil
- 100 ml of vegetable stock
- salt
- pepper
- ½ dried thyme
- ½ bunch chives (10 g)
- One organic lemon

Preparation

- Rinse the fish fillets, pat dry and drizzle with 2 tbsps. lemon juice. Clean leeks, wash and cut into rings.

- Heat 1 tbsps. Oil in a pan, dab fish dry, sauté for 2 minutes at medium heat. Then turn over, add the remaining lemon juice and 50 ml of vegetable stock and cover, cook for 5-7 minutes on low heat.

- Meanwhile, heat remaining oil in a saucepan, sauté the leek rings in medium heat for 2 minutes, season with salt, pepper, and thyme. Add remaining vegetable stock and cook the leek for 5 minutes over low heat.

- Meanwhile, wash chives, shake dry and cut into small rolls. Rinse lemon hot and cut into quarters.

- Season fish fillets and leeks with salt and pepper, arrange on plates and garnish with chives and lemon quarters.

91. Grilled Meatball Recipe
24 pieces

Preparation time: 30 minutes

Cooking time: 15 minutes

Ingredients

600 grams of medium-fat ground beef (beef-sheep mixed)

1 slice of stale bread

1 small onion bulb

1 egg

1 teaspoon of cumin

1/2 teaspoon of salt

1/2 teaspoon black pepper

Preparation

1. The meatballs you prepare, in the refrigerator and in a closed container for at least 2 hours until you add non-stick eggs and delicious meatballs you can prepare.

2. Cooking Suggestions for Grilled Meatball Recipe
3. You can add the finely chopped parsley to the meatball mortar according to your desire.
4. How to make Grilled Meatball Recipe?
5. Take 600 grams of medium fat ground beef into the mixing bowl. Add 1 egg, 1 grated nectarine, 1 slice of stale bread, 1 teaspoon of cumin, half teaspoon of salt and pepper.
6. Add all the ingredients to the consistency of the meatball mortar, knead until it is recovered and close the stretch film and let it rest in the refrigerator for at least half an hour.

7. Cut walnut-sized pieces of meatball mortar

8. Give the meatballs flat with your hands moistened with water.

9. Index the meatballs to the hot pan where you grease.

10. Start cooking by inverting. Continue this process until all the meatballs are cooked.

11. Your meatballs are ready; you can serve hot and hot. Enjoy your meal.

92. Chicken Recipe with Sauce

For 4 people

20 minutes

Cooking time: 20 minutes

Ingredients

800 grams of fillet chicken breast

2 tablespoons olive oil

1 tomato

1 clove of garlic

1 small onion bulb

1 teaspoon tomato paste

1 teaspoon hot sauce (or 1/2 teaspoon powdered red pepper)

1 teaspoon of oregano

1 teaspoon of coriander (if desired)

1/4 teaspoon cumin

Preparation

Tip of Chicken Recipe with Sauce

1. If you have time to extend the marination period of chicken meat in the sauce mixture you prepare, leave for 1 hour in the refrigerator.
2. Chicken Recipe Cooking Suggestion
3. You can also cook the chicken with sauce on the grill or pan on greasy paper.

4. Chicken Recipe How to Make?
5. Cut the breasts of fillet chicken which you wash in water and dry with paper towel into long thin strips.
6. For the sauce mixture; After peeling the skin, drain the juice of the onion you planed. You can use the posa portion for another meal.
7. Grate the tomato with the thin portion of the grater. Put the onion juice and grated tomatoes in a deep mixing bowl.
8. Mix with olive oil, grated garlic, tomato paste, hot sauce, thyme, cumin and coriander.
9. Take the chopped fillet chicken breasts into the mixing bowl and cover them and leave them in the refrigerator.
10. For long periods of rest (at least one hour and one night if you have time), pass the chicken meat horizontally to the wooden skewers.
11. Cook as soon as possible by inverting the duplex on a pre-heated pan or grill.

12. According to desire; Share with your loved ones on heated lavash with the addition of curly lettuce leaves, ring-cut red onions and tomato slices.

93. Liver Shish Recipe

4 people

Preparation time: 30 minutes

Cooking time: 20 minutes

Ingredients

1 kilogram of lamb gras

300 grams of tail oil

1 teaspoon of salt

1/2 teaspoon of cumin

For Shuttle:

2 medium onions

1 teaspoon sumac

Preparation

1. After washing with plenty of water and draining the excess water, cut the lamb liver into small pieces with the help of paper towels. Blend with salt.
2. Cut the tail fat to match the lungs. Start moving the liver parts to the garbage skewers. Insert two or three parts of the liver followed by a piece of tail oil. Do the same on all the bottles.
3. Turn the liver skewers upside down in the barbecue and cook all over until golden.
4. Serve with hot cumin sprinkled yufka breads on the hot plates served in the liver skewers, chopping after chopping the sumac and dry onions served with the onions.

Service Suggestion of Liver Recipe

You can chop dry bulbs, sauté on high heat, season with spices and serve with liver skewer.

94. Vegetable lasagna

For 4 people:

Ingredients

80 g Puy lentils

4 tbsp. olive oil + a little to coat the vegetables

1 tomato Coarse chopped beef heart

1 minced garlic clove

1 diced beetroot

1/2 tsp. tamari (soy sauce)

1 tbsp. dehydrated shallot dehydrated

1 pinch powdered cumin

400 g butternut squash cut into thin slices

300 g zucchini thinly sliced in length

Preparation:

1. Preheat the oven to temperature 170 ° C (Th 5-6). Put the lentils inside a small saucepan and cover them with water. Boil it and cook for 10 to 15 minutes until al dente. Drain and reserve.

2. Meanwhile, heat the oil inside a large saucepan, then crush the tomato that will be the base of the sauce. Add garlic and beetroot, tamari, shallot, and cumin. Pour 2 tablespoons of water and cook for 15 minutes over medium heat to obtain a thick puree. Add the lentils to the contents of the pan, add a little more water and simmer for another 5 minutes.

3. Spread half of the butternut and one-third of the zucchini in a baking dish, then cover with half of the lentil sauce. Repeat the same process and finish with a layer of zucchini. Spread them over with olive oil and cook for 45 minutes, until the vegetables are just tender.

You can replace olive oil with parsley oil.

Nutritional Facts

Calories 65

% Daily Value*

Total Fat 0.2 g   0%

Saturated fat 0 g   0%

Polyunsaturated fat 0.1 g

Monounsaturated fat 0 g

Cholesterol 0 mg   0%

Sodium 35 mg   1%

Potassium 169 mg   4%

Total Carbohydrate 13 g   4%

Dietary fiber 4.4 g   17%

Sugar 3.1 g

Protein 2.9 g   5%

95. Broccoli and lentils salad

Ingredients for 4 people

4 cup dried lentils,

2 onions,

4 bay leaves,

 4 broccolis divided into florets,

4 grated carrot,

Olive oil,

4 clove of garlic,

4 tablespoon of balsamic vinegar,

4 lemons,

 Salt, and pepper

Preparation

4. Our first step will be to cook the
    lentils. To do this, once washed,
    place them in the pressure cooker

together with a liter of water, 1/4 onion, bay leaves, a spoonful of salt and a tablespoon of olive oil, cover and count 8 minutes later that the pot has reached its pressure point. If we do not have an electric pressure cooker, it will be enough to put them to boil inside a covered pan for 30 minutes. Once cooked, drain and reserve.

5. While the lentils are cooking, we blanch the broccoli. Nothing is as simple as dipping the broccoli florets in boiling water for three minutes, then drain and immerse another three minutes in ice water. Next, we prepare vinaigrette with lemon juice, crushed garlic, balsamic vinegar, salt and pepper to taste.

6. Once the lentils and broccoli are cooked, and the carrot is grated, we proceed to assemble our salad. The secret of this one, in particular, is to give flavor to the lentils, reason why we will place them in a bowl, and we will bathe them with the vinaigrette, trying that they are covered

completely; Let them rest like this for two minutes and then integrate the carrot and broccoli florets, stir and serve immediately.

Tasting

This fresh salad of broccoli and lentils is a recipe that has a very good balance both in texture and flavor.

The softness of the lentils contrasts with the crunchy texture of the carrot and broccoli, while the strong flavor of garlic, and then balsamic vinegar is softened by the acidity of the lemon and the sweetness of the carrot. To serve it, we will not need more than a glass of fresh water and enough time and attention to enjoy it.

Nutritional Facts

Calories: 5.8

% Daily Value

Total fat 0.0g 0.0%

Saturated Fat 0.0g 0.0%

Trans Fat 0.0g

Cholesterol 0.0mg 0.0%

Sodium 4.2mg 0.0%

Total Carbs 0.8g 0.3%

Dietary Fiber 0.7g 2.6%

Sugars 0.0g

Protein 0.3g

Vitamin A 1.6%

Vitamin C 10.0%

Calcium 1.0%

Iron 0.7%

96. Waldorf salad with pineapple

Preparation: 30 min

Finished in 1 h 30 min

Ingredients

For 4 portions

3 bars

Celery (about 200 g)

1lemon

1 piece celeriac (about 200 g)

2 small red-skinned apples (approx. 100 g each)

1 tbsp.

Walnut kernels

2 tbsps.

Salad cream

5 tbsps.

Milk (1.5% fat)

White pepper

150 g

Fresh pineapple (pulp)

Preparation

1. Wash celery, clean, remove if necessary and set the tender green aside. Cut the celery into small cubes and place in a bowl.
2. Halve lemon and squeeze. Peel celeriac, wash and grate coarsely. Add to the celery and mix with 3 tablespoons of lemon juice.
3. Wash apples, dry, quarter and core. Cut into small columns or cubes. Give to the celery.
4. Roughly chop walnuts. Smooth the salad cream with the milk and season with pepper.
5. Mix the salad cream with the celery-apple mixture and the nuts.
6. Finely chop the celery green and bring it under the salad. Cover the salad covered for at least 1 hour cold.

To serve, cut the pineapple into small pieces and lift it under the salad — season with lemon juice and pepper to taste.

Nutritional Facts

Calories: 99 kcal

97. High-protein pizza cabbage with Nutri-Plus

Ingredients

200 g   spelt flour

60ml   Nutri-Plus Protein Powder Neutral

200 ml of water

10ml   baking powder

100 ml Sieved tomatoes

1 tbsp. mixed herbs

80ml   colorful paprika

30ml   mushrooms

30ml   peas

20ml   olives

1 spring onion

Smoothing   Salt, pepper, paprika

Preparation

Preparation time: 30 minutes

Makes 4 pizza buffets

1.   Preheat the oven to 180 ° C.

2.   Put the spilled flour, the protein powder, the baking powder and a pinch of salt in a bowl and mix everything thoroughly.

3.   Now add the water and knead the mass into a firm dough.

4.   Divide the dough into 4 pieces to form flat baguettes.

5.   Place the baguettes on the baking sheet lined and the baking paper and bake for about 5 minutes.

6.   In time you take care of the surface. Mix the tomato with herbs and spices and cut the vegetables into small cubes.

7.   Remove the pre-baked baguettes from the oven, sprinkle with the tomato sauce and spread the toppings on top.

8.   Bake the pizza cabbies for another 10 minutes until they are nicely brown and crispy.

Nutritional Facts

Calories   339.9

Total Fat   15.9 g

Saturated Fat   1.7 g

Polyunsaturated Fat   10.4 g

Monounsaturated Fat   2.5 g

Cholesterol   136.8 mg

Sodium   162.3 mg

Potassium   565.7 mg

Total Carbohydrate   20 g

Dietary Fiber   6.6 g

Sugars   0.0 g

Protein   24.2 g

98. Smoked Salmon Stuffed With Russian Salad

For 4 person

Ingredients:

500 g of smoked salmon

4 potatoes

4 carrots

200 g of frozen peas

200 g of green beans

6 eggs

400 ml of soft olive oil

5 lemon

Salt and pepper

12 sheets of romaine lettuce

Chive

Preparation

1. Cook the vegetables from the salad. Peel the carrots and the potatoes, wash them and cut them into cubes. Wash, blunt and chop the green beans. Boil the carrots in plenty of salt water for 15 minutes. Add the potatoes and cook them for seven more minutes. Add the green beans, and then continue cooking another 3 minutes. Finally, add the peas, cook five more minutes and drain all the vegetables.

2. Boil the eggs and make the mayonnaise. On the one hand, cook two eggs 10 minutes in salt water. Refresh them, peel them and chop them. And on the other, beat the remaining egg with the juice of half a lemon, salt, and pepper, and then add the oil, in a thread and beat until you get a thick mayonnaise.

3. Make the salad and stuff the salmon. First, mix the cooked vegetables and the chopped hard-boiled eggs with the mayonnaise. And stir until they are well incorporated. And then,

distribute the salad in the salmon slices and roll them up.

4. Assemble the plate and serve. Finally, wash and drain the lettuce. Cut it into julienne and break it into four plates. Arrange the rolls over it, and serve them sprinkled with the chopped chives.

Nutritional Facts

Calories   169.6

Total Fat   8.5 g

Saturated Fat   4.6 g

Cholesterol   34.0 mg

Sodium   723.8 mg

Potassium   104.7 mg

Total Carbohydrate   6.7 g

Dietary Fiber   2.9 g

Sugars   1.3 g

Protein   16.5 g

99. Salad with asparagus, cherry tomatoes, and cottage cheese

For 4 person

Ingredients:

4 bunches of green asparagus

250 g of cherry tomatoes

100 g of cottage cheese

60 g peeled walnuts

60 g of kikos (toasted corn)

40 g of peeled sunflower seeds

4 tablespoons of vinegar

6 tablespoons of olive oil

Pepper and salt

Preparation

1. Clean the asparagus. First, wash the asparagus under the stream of cold water, remove the hardest part of the

stem, and cut them into pieces of the same size.

2. Put water to boil and cook. While preparing the asparagus, boil plenty of salt water in a casserole, add them and cook for 10 minutes till they are tender but whole.

3. Interrupting the cooking. Once they are done, then remove them with a slotted spoon and immerse them for a few moments in a bowl of ice water to halt cooking. In this way, they will maintain their intense green color. And then, drain them again to eliminate all the water.

4. Prepare the rest of the ingredients. Wash the tomatoes, dry them with absorbent paper and cut them in half. Drain the cottage cheese and crumble it. And cut the nuts into small pieces.

5. Make the vinaigrette. Arrange the vinegar in a bowl. Add a pinch of salt, pepper, and pour the oil, little by little, continuing to beat with a fork, until you get well-emulsified vinaigrette.

6. Emulator and serve. Distribute the asparagus in four bowls. Add the tomatoes, the crumbled cottage cheese, and the chopped walnuts. Dress with the previous vinaigrette. And decorate with sunflower seeds and chopped kikos.

Nutritional Facts

Calories   302.2

Total Fat   10.8 g

Saturated Fat   1.9 g

Cholesterol   58.4 mg

Sodium   618.0 mg

Potassium   601.9 mg

Total Carbohydrate   10.0 g

Dietary Fiber   3.1 g

Sugars   2.2 g

Protein   37.5 g

100.   Mussels with Butter and Indian Touch

Ingredients

for two people: 20 mussels of good size,

80 g of butter,

2 spoonful of curry powder,

 salt, and chopped chives.

For 4 person

Preparation:

We clean the mussels under the tap, rubbing the outside to remove adhesions and stones and removing the beards that appear. We put them to the fire with 50 ml of water, in a covered casserole, until they open. It will not take more than 7 minutes. Once ready, remove the mussels from the pan and finish opening them, forcing the shell and removing one of the two. We place them in the source in which we will serve them. Inside a medium pan, melt the butter, add the curry and stir. Pour over the mussels and then decorate with chopped chives.

Nutritional Facts

Calories 9   % Daily Values

Total Fat 0.22g   0%

Saturated Fat 0.042g   0%

Polyunsaturated Fat 0.061g

Monounsaturated Fat 0.051g

Cholesterol 3mg   1%

Total Carbohydrate 0.37g   0%

Dietary Fiber 0g   0%

Sugars 0g

Protein 1.19g

101. Keto fried chicken with butter and broccoli

Portion: 4 people

Ingredients

650 g boneless chicken thighs

150 g butter

450 g broccoli

½ leek

1 tsp. garlic powder

Salt and ground black pepper Ingredients

650 g boneless chicken thighs

150 g butter

450 g broccoli

½ leek

1 tsp. garlic powder

Salt and ground black pepper

Preparation

Fry the chicken in the air fryer over medium heat for about 3-5 minutes on each side, depending on the thickness. Pepper generously.

Make sure the chicken is cooked. Lower the heat and then cook another minute if you are not sure.

Remove the chicken from the air fryer and cover it with aluminum foil or put it on low heat in the air fryer to keep it warm.

Rinse, and then trim the broccoli, including the stem. Cut into pieces. Cut the leek into thick slices.

Fry the vegetables at medium heat in the air fryer you used for the chicken. Add more garlic powder and mix pepper.

Serve chicken and vegetables with a good dose of butter on top.

Advice!

This dish can be varied infinitely. Do not hesitate to experiment with various condiments, both for chicken. If you prefer to serve it with a spreadable sauce, try mixing the sauce with mayonnaise to your liking to add a spicy touch.

Nutritional Information

Calories   176.6

Total Fat   2.0 g

Saturated Fat   0.5 g

Cholesterol   68.4 mg

Sodium   698.4 mg

Potassium   678.9 mg

Total Carbohydrate 8.4 g

Dietary Fiber   4.3 g

Sugars   2.3 g

Protein   32.3 g

102. Vegan vegetable kebabs with herbs

Vegan vegetable skewers with herbs are the perfect alternative for those who want to barbecue meatless or even look for a delicious vegetable garnish.

Port: 4

Time: 30 min

Ingredients

400 g cherry tomatoes

200 g of zucchini

200 g of radish

200 g paprika

200 g mushrooms

2 onions

2 sprig of rosemary

4 sprigs of thyme

6 tbsp. olive oil

Colorful pepper

Sea-salt

Preparation

1. Wash the tomatoes, curettes and radishes and drain

- Cut the zucchini into thick slices and divide into 4 pieces
- Free the radish from the green and cut in half
- For peppers, remove the cores and partitions, rinse and cut into pieces.

2. Peel the onion and cut into pieces

- Wash the herbs and shake them dry, then pluck the leaves from the stalk and chop
- Clean the mushrooms and cut off the dry stem end
- Then cut the mushrooms in half.

3. Place the prepared ingredients alternately on wooden skewers

- Place the skewers on a plate and then drizzle with oil
- Season with salt, pepper and sprinkle with the herbs
- Grill skewers all around on the hot grill or in the grill pan.

103. **Savory Chicken Thighs with** Grill Marinade

Cooking time: 30 to 60 min

Ingredients

Servings: 4

One toe garlic (crushed)

1 tablespoon mustard

4 tsps. sugar (brown)

2 teaspoon chili powder

Pepper (black, freshly ground)

2 tbsps. olive oil

10 pcs chicken lower leg

Preparation

1. For the spicy chicken legs with grill marinade, mix the garlic with the mustard, the brown sugar, the chili powder, a pinch of salt and freshly ground pepper. Mix with the oil.
2. Rub in the chicken thighs with the marinade and marinate for 20 minutes.
3. Put the chicken thighs in the basket and push the basket into the Pressure cooker. Set the timer to 10-12 minutes.
4. Fry the chicken thighs at 200 ° C until brown. Minimize the temperature to 150 ° C and fry the chicken thighs for another 10 minutes until they are cooked.
5. The spicy chicken leg with barbecue marinade with corn salad and baguette serve.

104. Organic grilled asparagusrecipe

Preparation time: 5 minutes

Cooking time: 5 minutes

Yield: 4 servings

Ingredients

2 pound of asparagus

2 tbsps. buttered with grass (melted)

Unrefined sea salt

Pepper to taste

Preparation:

1. Cut asparagus, this is easily accomplished by breaking off the ends where it naturally breaks off.

2. Pour the melted butter over the asparagus and toss for coating.

3. Season generously with salt and pepper.

4. Place on a hot grill (medium heat) and grill for about 5-10 minutes until the asparagus is soft (turn frequently).

105.   California Chicken

Yields: 4 servings

Preparation time: 20 minutes

Total time: 40 minutes

Ingredients

3/4 c. balsamic vinegar

1 teaspoon. Garlic Powder

2 tbsp. honey

2 tbsp. extra virgin olive oil

2 tsps. Italian spice

Kosher salt

Freshly ground black pepper

4 boneless chicken breast without skin

4 slices of mozzarella

4 slices of avocado

4 tomato slices

2 tbsp. Freshly cut basil for garnish

Balsamic glaze for drizzling

Preparation

1. In a small bowl whisk balsamic vinegar, add garlic powder, honey, oil and Italian spices and season with salt and the pepper. Pour the chicken and marinate for 20 minutes.

2. When you are ready to grill, heat the grill to medium high. Grate the oil grills and chicken until charred and cooked through, 8 minutes each side.

3. Top chicken with the mozzarella, avocado and tomato and lid grill melt, 2 minutes.

4. Garnish with basil and then drizzle with some balsamic glaze.

106. Coriander lime Grilledsalmon

Yields: 4

Preparation time: 0 hours 5 minutes

Total time: 0 hours 25 minutes

Ingredients

4 (6 ounces) salmon fillets

Kosher salt

Freshly ground black pepper

4 tbsp. butter

1/2 c. lime juice

1/4 c. honey

2 garlic cloves, chopped

2 TBSP. Chopped coriander

Preparation

1. Season salmon with salt and pepper. Heat the grill and place the salmon meat side down on the grill. Cook for 8 minutes, then turn and cook on the other side until the salmon is cooked through, another 6 minutes. Let rest for 5 minutes.

2. In the meantime, prepare the sauce: inside a medium saucepan over medium the heat, add butter, lime juice, honey and the garlic. Mix it until butter is melted and all ingredients are combined. Turn off heat and add cilantro.

3. Pour salmon over sauce and serve.

107.   **Grilled Plums with Orange,**
Vanilla, and Pistaches
Preparation time: 10 minutes

Cooking time: 30 minutes

Ingredients

2 Servings

1/2 cup chopped brown sugar, for honey

1/3 cup of water for honey

2 pieces of star anise, for honey

1/2 piece of a cinnamon slit for honey

1/8 teaspoon of clove powder for honey

4 pieces of a plum cut in half, without bone

1/4 cup of well-grated coconut

Preparation

1. Preheat the oven to 180 ° C.

2. Heat the pot on high heat with the brown sugar and water, add the star anise, the cinnamon stick with the clove powder, and reduce the preparation to form honey.
3. In a baking dish add the plums and bathe with honey. Cook for 30 minutes until the taste of honey is impregnated with plums and softened.
4. Serve and decorate with anise and grated coconut.

108.   Grilled Ox Hearts

Ingredients

2 Ox hearts or big meat tomatoes

2 Mozzarella di Bufala

2 1TL sugar

Salt

Pepper

Ingredients:

Pesto Genovese

1.2 clove of garlic

100ml olive oil

5G pine nuts

30G Basil (corresponds to about two pots)

50G Parmesan

Black pepper

One anchovy

One lemon

Preparation

1. Pound pesto in a mortar or use hand blender. Rasp cheese. Use only the basil leaves.
2. Finely chop all ingredients. First, process the dry

ingredients into a fine paste, and then add the olive oil and anchovy.

3. Season the pesto with salt and pepper. To preserve the color for longer, add some fresh lemon juice.

Preparing ox hearts

4. Cut the tomatoes to 2 cm thick slices. Salt on both sides and lightly sugar.

5. Cut the mozzarella into thin slices.

6. Preheat the grill. Alternatively, prepare at 220° top/bottom heat in the oven.

7. Grill tomatoes for 20 minutes on medium heat, turn after 10 minutes. When the tomatoes are almost done, cover with cheese and cook for 5 minutes until the cheese has melted.

8. Peppers, serve immediately with pesto.

109.   Avocado wrapped in bacon

Cooking time: 15 to 30 min

Servings: 4

Ingredients

2 avocados (ripe)

15-20 strips of bacon

Preparation

1. For the avocado wrapped in bacon wrapped in bacon, first, preheat the oven to 180 ° C. Cover a baking tray with baking paper.
2. Halve the avocado and remove the kernel. Carefully remove the pulp (preferably with a tablespoon). Then cut lengthwise into approximately 1 cm thick slits.
3. Wrap each column with a strip of bacon and place on the baking sheet.

Put the avocado wrapped in bacon in the oven for about 15 minutes until the bacon is crispy. Best observe because every oven is a little different.

Tip

The bacon-wrapped avocado is ideal as a starter, snack, or side dish. It can also be prepared as a grill on the grill.

110.   Lettuce Tacos with Chickento the Shepherd

Preparation time: 1 h 20 minutes

Cooking time: 35 minutes

6 Servings

Ingredients

50 grams of achiote for the marinade

1/4 cup of apple vinegar for the marinade

3 pieces of guajillo chile clean, deveined and seedless, hydrated for the marinade

2 pieces of wide chili clean, deveined and seedless, hydrated for the marinade

3 garlic cloves for the marinade

1/4 piece of white onion for the marinade

1/2 cup pineapple juice for marinade

1 tablespoon salt marinade

1 tablespoon fat pepper for marinade

2 pieces of clove for the marinade

1 tablespoon oregano for the marinade

1 piece of roasted guaje tomato, for the marinade

1 tablespoon cumin for the marinade

1 piece of boneless and skinless chicken breast, cut into small cubes

1 tablespoon of olive or flax oil

Enough of French Lettuce Eva

1/2 piece of pineapple cut into half moons

1/2 cup chopped coriander

1/2 cup finely chopped purple onion

To the taste of tree chili sauce to accompany

To the taste of lemon to accompany

Preparation

1. For the marinade, blend the achiote, vinegar, chilies, garlic, onion, juice, salt, pepper, cloves, oregano, tomato, and cumin until a homogeneous mixture is obtained.
2. Put the chicken and the marinade inside a bowl with the shepherd marinade for 1 hour in refrigeration.
3. Heat a pan over medium heat with the oil and cook the chicken you marinated until it is cooked. Reserve covered.
4. Heat a grill over high heat, roast the pineapple until golden brown, remove and cut into cubes, reserve.

5. On a table place sheets of French Lettuce Eva®, add the chicken to the shepherd and serve with the roasted pineapple, cilantro, onion, served with a little sauce and lemons.

Nutritional information

Percentage of daily values based on a 2,000-calorie diet.

Calories   92.2   kcal 4.6%

Carbohydrates   22.3   g 7.4%

Proteins   1.6   g 3.2%

Lipids   0.9   g 1.3%

Dietary fiber   2.9   g 5.8%

Sugars   6.6   g 7.4%

Cholesterol   0.0   mg 0.0%

111.   Colorful Vegetable Strudel

Cooking time: 30 to 60 min

Servings: 2

Ingredients

For the vegetable strudel:

- 1 pkg of puff pastry
- 1/2 head of broccoli
- 3 carrots
- 1/2 head of caramel
- 1 bell pepper (red)
- 2 garlic cloves
- Caraway (ground)
- salt
- Pepper (from the mill)
- 1 egg (to brush)
- 1 onion For the Béchamel sauce:
- 50 g of butter
- 50 g of flour
- 250 ml of milk For the herb sauce:
- 1 pinch of nutmeg (ground)
- 200 g of yogurt
- 125 g sour cream
- 1/2 bunch chives
- 1/2 bunch of parsley
- some dill (fresh)

- salt
- pepper

Preparation:

1. For the colorful vegetable strudel from the Air fryer first or you use an oven, wash the vegetables, clean and cut into bite-sized pieces. Brew in boiling salted water for about 2 minutes. Drain well.
2. Peel garlic including the onions and cut into small cubes.
3. For the béchamel sauce, melt the butter, adding first the flour and then the milk, stirring constantly. Add garlic, onion, vegetables, salt, pepper and cumin.
4. Roll out the puff pastry and then put the stuffing on the lower third. Beat in the sides and roll up the dough to a firm vortex.
5. Whisk the egg and brush the whirlpool with it.
6. Bake for approximately 25 minutes at 180 ° C in the Air Fryer.

In the meantime, prepare the herb sauce. For chopped chives, parsley and dill finely. Stir all Ingredients until smooth and season the sauce.

Serve vegetable strudel from the hot air fryer with herb sauce. Colorful vegetable strudel from the Air fryer also tastes cold.

Nutritional Information:

Calories 286.6

Total Fat 8.6 g

Saturated Fat 2.5 g

Polyunsaturated Fat 1.5 g

Monounsaturated Fat 2.5 g

Cholesterol 48.2 mg

Sodium 916.3 mg

Potassium 362.4 mg

Total Carbohydrate 37.5 g

Dietary Fiber 6.7 g

Sugars 2.5 g

Protein 15.8 g

112.   Creamy Strawberry cup

For one person

Preparation time: 10 mins

Freezing time: 30 mins

To make this delicious ice cream we need:

Ingredients:

- 500 gr of very ripe raspberries
- 25 cl of cooking cream
- 235 gr of sugar

Preparation:

All you have to do put all the ingredients in the blender, and we are going to beat it little by little until you achieve the desired texture, and then put it in the freezer in a silicone mold, leave it in at least 30 minutes.

Nutritional Information

- 20% Total Fat 13g
- 41% Saturated Fat 8.2g.
- Trans Fat 0g
- 18% Cholesterol 53mg
- 4% Sodium 96mg
- 7% Potassium 262mg
- 10% Total Carbohydrates 30g
- 7% Dietary Fiber 1.8g

113.   Apple Green Ceviche

3 Servings

Preparation time: 10 minutes

Cooking time: 20 minutes

Ingredients

- 1/4 cup of lemon juice
- 1/3 cup of orange juice
- 2 tablespoons of olive oil
- 1/4 bunch of cilantro

- 2 pieces of green apple without peel, cut into medium cubes
- 1 piece of finely chopped serrano chili
- 1 cup of jicama cut into medium cubes
- 1 piece of avocado cut into cubes
- 1 cup cucumber cut into cubes
- 1/4 bunch of finely chopped basil leaf
- 1/4 cup of finely chopped cilantro
- 1 pinch of salt
- 1 piece of sliced radish
- 1 piece of serrano chili cut into slices
- 1/4 piece of purple onion

Preparation

1. Add lemon juice, orange juice, olive oil and cilantro to the blender. Blend perfectly well. Reservation.
2. Add to a bowl the apple, serrano pepper, jicama, avocado, cucumber, basil, cilantro, mix with the

preparation of the blender and season perfectly well.

3. Serve the ceviche in a deep dish and decorate with the radish the chile serrano and the purple onion. Enjoy

Nutritional information

- Percentage of daily values based on a 2,000-calorie diet.
- Calories   61.9   kcal 3.1%
- Carbohydrates   14.4   g 4.8%
- Proteins   1.6   g 3.1%
- Lipids   0.3   g 0.4%
- Dietary fiber   5.1   g 10%
- Sugars   6.2   g 6.9%
- Cholesterol   0.0   mg 0.0%

114.   Vegetable and Kale Soup

Preparation time: 10 minutes

Cooking time: 30 minutes

Ingredients

2 Servings

2 tablespoons of olive oil

1/2 piece of white onion filleted

1 celery stick cut in cubes

1 cup chopped pore

1 tablespoon finely chopped garlic

1 cup sliced mushrooms

1 cup mushroom filleted

2 cups of kale

1/2 piece of fennel the bulb, cut into sticks

6 cups of beef broth

1 pinch of salt

1 pinch of pepper

1/4 cup of almond

Preparation

1. Heat a medium deep pot over medium heat, add the olive oil, onion and celery until they release the aroma, add the pore, garlic and mushrooms with the mushrooms until they start to release the juice, add the kale until I soften with the fennel. Cook for 5 more minutes.
2. Fill with the beef broth and season to your liking. Cook until it boils, covering it to prevent it from evaporating.
3. Serve in a bowl with a little fresh kale at the end and sliced almonds. Enjoy

Nutritional information

Calories 507 kcal 25%

Carbohydrates 65.6 g 22%

Proteins 35.8 g 72%

Lipids 16.3 g 25%

Sugars 10.7 g 12%

Cholesterol 0.0 mg 0.0%

115. Salad with tahini sauce

6 People

Preparation Time 30 Min

Ingredients

4 carrots

1 cucumber

1 long pink radish

2 fresh onions

1 handful of arugula

1 black radish

For the sauce

1 tablespoon (s) of tahini

3 tablespoon (s) of olive oil

1 lemon

1 clove of garlic

1 small piece of ginger

10 sprigs of coriander

Chili pepper

Freshly ground pepper

Preparation

1. Peel the carrots, black radish, cucumber, onions, ginger, and garlic clove. Wash the pink radish, the arugula, the leafless coriander. Wring the arugula and dry the coriander.

2. Finely grate all the vegetables. Slice the onions. Chop the garlic. Grate the ginger.

3. Gather the vegetables, onions, and arugula in a salad bowl.

4.For the sauce: pour the tahiné, the oil, the lemon juice, the chopped garlic, the grated ginger, salt, pepper, one pinch of chili, and the chopped cilantro in a jar with a lid. Add 2 tsp. About water, close, shake the jar well to combine the ingredients, and pour over the salad.

116.   Vegan bowl

An all-in-one dish made up of cereals, legumes, vegetable proteins and vegetables.

4 People

Preparation Time: 45 Mins

Cooking Time: 40 Mins

Ingredients

250 g of pea's raw chick

4 red onions

3 cloves of garlic

1 bunch basil, chopped

1 g smoked paprika

3 carrots

2 zucchini

2 g garam masala

500 g cooked semi-whole rice

500 g red cabbage

1/2 glass (s) of white vinegar

1.5 cucumbers

200 g of yogurt to soy

2 lemons yellow

1 bunch of chopped mint

Salt pepper

Olive oil

100 g baby spinach

Preparation

1. Soak the chickpeas the day before in a large amount of water. The next day, drain them and then dry them well.

2. Mix the chickpeas with 1 onion, 1 clove of garlic and the chopped basil. Salt, pepper and add the paprika. Form walnut-sized balls and place them on a baking sheet. Put the falafels in the oven for 20 minutes at 180 ° C (th. 6). Halfway through cooking, turn them over.

3. Brown the sliced carrots and zucchini with 2 tbsp. olive oil, 2 cloves of garlic and 2 chopped onions. Season it with salt, including pepper and add the garam masala. Cook for 10 minutes to keep the vegetables firm. Add the rice and leave for another 5 minutes over low heat.

4. Cut the red cabbage with a mandolin, sprinkle it with vinegar. Let stand for 10 minutes.

5. Cut 1 cucumber in half lengthwise. Remove the seeds. Grate it and set aside. Add the yogurt, 1 chopped onion, the juice of the 2 lemons, the mint, 1 tsp. olive oil, salt and pepper.

6. Serve the rice with vegetables in bowls, topped with the yogurt sauce, falafels, red cabbage, the rest of the chopped cucumber and baby spinach.

117. Thai Pumpkin Soup

For two persons

Preparation: 10 mins.

Cooking time: 15 mins

Creamy pumpkin soup with a hint of Thailand: coconut milk, ginger, and chili.

Ingredients

- 3EL Coconut Oil
- 500G Pumpkin
- 400G Carrots
- 1piece Spring Onion (50 G)
- 1piece Small Chili
- 1piece Clove Of Garlic
- 5cm Ginger (30 G)
- 1TL Turmeric
- 500ml Vegetable Stock
- 400ml Coconut Milk
- 5leaves Thai Basil
- 1piece Lime Leaf
- Prize Salt
- EL Soy Sauce
- Heap Spoon Of Coconut Oil
- Prize Black Pepper
- 1EL Lime Juice
- Fresh coriander to serve

Preparation

1. Cut off the pumpkin drink. Peel pumpkin as needed hollow out the pumpkin and weigh it. Use the same amount of carrots. Peel carrots. Cut pumpkin and carrots into large

pieces. Peel ginger and turmeric. Finely chop the spring onion, chili, ginger, turmeric, and garlic.
2. Heat coconut oil in a saucepan. Fry spring onion, ginger, chili, turmeric, and garlic. Add carrots and pumpkin and roast without browning. Add soup and coconut milk, add basil and lime leaf. Bring to a boil, add basil and lime leaf. Simmer on a flame for about 15 minutes until the vegetables are tender. Prick vegetables with a needle. If the vegetables slip off easily, it is soft.
3. Remove lime leaf and basil. Puree the soup with a hand blender.
4. Season it with salt, pepper, soy sauce, and lime juice. Serve with a little coriander.

Nutritional Information

- Calories 161.7 % Daily Value
- Total Fat 12.4g   -
- Saturated fat 10.8g   -
- Carbohydrates 11.3g -
- Net carbs 8.8g -
- Sugar 2.6g   -
- Fiber 2.5g   11%
- Protein 4.5g

118.   Forgotten Vegetable Soup

A recipe from my grandmother, which has always been so successful! (Lolita André)

4 People

Preparation Time: 20 Min.

Cooking Time: 55 Mins

Ingredients

600 g Jerusalem artichokes

400 g parsnips

1 kg of butternut squash

500 g carrots

2 red onions

3 cloves of garlic

1 sprig of thyme

1 tablespoon (s) of olive oil

1/2 teaspoon (s) of salt

Pepper

1 g smoked paprika

Preparation

1. Peel off and chop the onions and the garlic. Brown them with thyme and olive oil. Add salt, pepper and smoked paprika.

2. Peel the vegetables, rinse them and roughly cut them. Add them to the onions and sauté for 10 minutes.

3. Cover the vegetables with water and cook for 40 minutes.

4. Mix the soup using a food processor. Serve with seed crackers.

119.   Asparagus and trout salad

Excellent as a starter or main dish if you double the quantities.

4 people

Preparation time: 10 min.

Ingredients

400 g green asparagus

400 g raw skinless trout

40 g spring onions

100 g of young shoots (purslane, spinach...)

1 tablespoon (s) of caper flower

Vinaigrette

5 tablespoon (s) of olive oil

3 tablespoon (s) of apple cider vinegar

The juice of 1 lemon yellow

20 g spring onion whites

75 g capers

1/2 teaspoon (s) of salt

Preparation

1. Rinse and cut each asparagus lengthwise with a peeler to obtain strips. Place them in a colander and pour 2 l of boiling water over them, then immediately place them for 5 minutes in very cold water so that they retain a beautiful green color. Drain and set aside.

2. Cut the fish into 1 cm cubes.

3. Cut the green part of the onions into thin strips and soak them in water for a few minutes. Slice the white part and set aside.

4. Mix all ingredients for the dressing and mix in the blender.

5. Put the asparagus, the young shoots, and the white of the onions, the caper flowers and the raw fish in a bowl. Season with vinaigrette.

120.   Pumpkin and apple soup

Ingredients

- 450 grams (1 lb.) pumpkin
- 1 Granny Smith apple cored, and quartered
- One medium onion cut
- Two cloves garlic
- One tablespoon of olive oil
- salt
- ¼ teaspoon of cayenne more to taste
- 300 ml (1¼ cup) of vegetable stock
- freshly ground black pepper to add taste

- GARNISH:
- pomegranate arils
- some pumpkin seeds
- fresh parsley finely chopped

Preparation

1. Preheat the oven about 200 degrees C (or 392 degrees F). Line a large baking sheet with a parchment paper.
2. Cut the pumpkin half lengthways and scoop out seeds.

3. Slice each pumpkin half in half to make quarters and place, cut-side up, on a baking tray, along with the onions.
4. Drizzle with olive oil and then sprinkle some salt.
5. Bake for about 20 minutes, then add the garlic and apple, flip the pumpkin cut side down and then roast for another for 20 minutes, or until the flesh is soft.
6. Take a clean spoon to dip out the flesh of the pumpkin and transfer to a high-speed blender with the apple, onion, garlic (remove the skins), cayenne, and vegetable stock.
7. Blend on high for almost 2 minutes, or until silky smooth.
8. If too thick, add vegetable stock to thin it out and blend over. Taste and adjust the seasonings.
9. Serve, ladle soup into a bowl, and with pomegranate arils, pumpkin seeds, fresh parsley and freshly ground black pepper.
10. Then serve.
11. Refrigerate the leftovers inside an airtight container for 4 days.

121.   Vegetable casserole with cabbage

A veggie dish to let cook for a long time to increase all the flavors.

8 People

Preparation Time: 30 Min.

Cooking Time: 240 Mins

Calories: 398 Cal / Pers.

Ingredients

1 cabbage curly

1 small celeriac

6 apples earth bintje

4 carrots.4 turnip

4 raw beets

1 small cauliflower

1 heart of celery branch

3 sprigs of fresh thyme

3 bay leaves

1 tablespoon juniper berries

50 g butter

10 cl vegetable

4 tablespoon (s) of olive oil

Salt pepper

To serve

2 tablespoon (s) chopped parsley

Preparation

1. Trim the kale then take six green leaves and blanch them for 5 minutes in boiling salted water. Immerse them inside cold water and drain them. Cut the heart into 1 cm strips.

2. Peel the celeriac, potatoes, carrots, turnips and beets. Cut them into slices or slices 1 cm thick. Separate the florets from the cauliflower. Slice the celery stalk.

3. Brush a 28 cm diameter round cast iron casserole dish with half the oil. Line the inside with the blanched cabbage leaves, then divide all the vegetables in layers, sprinkling them with thyme, bay leaves, juniper berries, salt, pepper and hazelnuts. Fold down the cabbage leaves, brush them with the rest of the oil and add the broth.

4. Cover the casserole dish and place it in the oven at 150 ° C (th. 5). Cook it for 4 hours until the vegetables are tender and slightly caramelized.

5. Remove the casserole dish from the oven. Sprinkle with butter and chopped parsley. Serve immediately or warm.

122.   Vegetables soup

A basic of the kitchen.

6 people

Preparation time: 35 mins.

Cooking time: 100 MIN.

Ingredients

For 2 liters

.2 carrots

1 onion

4 shallots

1 white leek

1 celery branch

50 g celeriac

1/2 fennel

1 stick of lemongrass

1/2 bird's eye chili

.25 g fresh ginger

3 cloves of garlic

2 tablespoon (s) of olive oil

1/2 teaspoon ground black pepper

1/2 tablespoon coarse salt

4 cloves

1 star anise

1 bouquet garni

Preparation

1. Peel the vegetables. Cut the onion into quarters and then prick the cloves. Chop the shallots. Cut the carrots and celery stalks into sections. Cut the leek and ginger into slices. Slice the fennel. Coarsely chop the garlic cloves. Cut the lemongrass in half lengthwise. Remove the seeds from the bird's eye pepper.

2. Sweat all the ingredients in a saucepan with a little olive oil without letting them color. Add 2.5 l of water and simmer over

low heat for 1 h 30 min while foaming from time to time to remove the impurities.

123.   **Soup of noodles with**
vegetables

Quantity: 2 people

Preparation: 20 minutes

Cooking: 5 minutes

Ingredients:

2 liters of water

150 g of organic buckwheat noodles

2 cloves of garlic

1 laminated tender onion, including the tender green part

1 laminated leek

1 carrot cut in julienne

5 or 6 laminated mushrooms

1 trunk of celery, cut into thin slices

Half red pepper

Half green pepper

1 tbsp. fresh ginger

1 strip of wakame seaweed

1 pinch of sea salt

Ground black pepper

Extra virgin olive oil

Soy sauce

Parsley and chopped fresh chives sprinkle

Preparation:

1. In a pot with a lid, heat a tablespoon of oil and sauté the garlic, onion, and leek over medium heat.

2. Add the carrot, mushrooms, celery, and red and green pepper cut into thin strips, the freshly grated ginger, and the seaweed. Cover and sauté 3 to 4 minutes with the pot covered. If necessary add some tablespoon of water to facilitate cooking.

3. Salt, cover with water and boil on low heat for about 5 minutes.

4. In a separate pot, bring two liters of boiling water and boil the noodles (follow the package instructions).

5. Drain, immediately pour a small number of noodles into a bowl and add the broth with the vegetables.

6. Season with a string of soy sauce, sprinkle with the herbs and dress with a string of olive oil. Serves hot

Nutritional Information

Calories 159

% Daily Value

6%Total Fat 3.8g grams

9%Total Carbohydrates 26g grams

Sugars 4g grams

Protein 5.8g

124.　　Dry belly soup with cabbage and celery

The ingredients have the function of detoxifying the body, eliminating excess swelling and retention of liquid. Celery is diuretic, the onion has the function of detoxifying, the cabbage has low calories and improves bowel function, and the bell peppers bring satiety and more fiber to the body.

Ingredients:

1/2 chopped cabbage

6 large chopped onions

6 tomatoes chopped without seeds

3 stalks of celery

2 green peppers

Salt to taste

Pepper to taste

Oregano to taste

Preparation:

1. Wash vegetables and chop as instructed above. Bring all of these ingredients into a pan with water to cover.
2. Let it cook over medium-high heat with the pan semi-capped.
3. Season with salt, pepper and oregano and other spices and herbs you prefer.
4. Cook until the vegetables are tender. Serve immediately.

Nutritional Information

Calories: 165.2

Sugars: 4.1 g

Dietary Fiber: 12.0 g

Total Fat: 1.8 g

125.   Tomato and garlic soup

Quantity: 2 people

Preparation: 40 minutes

Cooking: 20 minutes

Ingredients:

Half a liter of water

1 purple onion, thinly sliced

8-10 cloves of garlic rolled

1 kilo of ripe tomatoes, without skin

2 or 3 bay leaves

1 pinch of cayenne pepper, optional for a spicier touch

1 pinch of black pepper

Sea salt, to taste

1 tsp. Provencal herbs

1 pinch of cumin to it sprinkle

Extra virgin olive oil

Preparation:

1. In a pot, sauté the onion and garlic in 1 tablespoon of olive oil. Remove often, so they do not burn.

2. Blanch the tomatoes into boiling water, remove the skin and, if you prefer, also the seeds.

3. Add to the pot the tomatoes cut in quarters and the rest of the ingredients. Remove and cook over low heat for 10 minutes and with the pot covered, until the tomato acquires a slightly orange tone.

4. Add the water, and boil for about 10 minutes.

5. Remove the bay leaves and crush until you get a light texture. If necessary, add more water and rectify salt.

6. Serve the hot soup dressed with a strand of extra virgin olive oil and sprinkled with the cumin. To learn more: "Help fight infections with the antibiotic power of garlic," explains nutritionist Llargués. It has traditionally been used to prevent infections. Its flavor is dominant, compensated in this recipe by the tomato.

Nutritional Information

Calories: 81.3

 Total Fat: 2.1 g

Dietary Fiber: 2.7 g

 Saturated Fat: 1.1 g

126.　　Apple Green Ceviche

Preparation time: 10 minutes

Cooking time: 20 minutes

Ingredients

3 Servings

   1/4 cup of lemon juice

   1/3 cup of orange juice

   2 tablespoons of olive oil

   1/4 bunch of cilantro

   2 pieces of green apple without peel, cut into medium cubes

1 piece of finely chopped serrano chili

1 cup of jicama cut into medium cubes

1 piece of avocado cut into cubes

1 cup cucumber cut into cubes

1/4 bunch of finely chopped basil leaf

1/4 cup of finely chopped cilantro

1 pinch of salt

1 piece of sliced radish

1 piece of serrano chili cut into slices

1/4 piece of purple onion

Preparation

4. Add lemon juice, orange juice, olive oil and cilantro to the blender. Blend perfectly well. Reservation.
5. Add to a bowl the apple, serrano pepper, jicama, avocado, cucumber, basil, cilantro, mix with the preparation of the blender and season perfectly well.

6. Serve the ceviche in a deep dish and decorate with the radish the chile serrano and the purple onion. Enjoy

Nutritional information

Calories   61.9   kcal 3.1%

Carbohydrates   14.4   g 4.8%

Proteins   1.6   g 3.1%

Lipids   0.3   g 0.4%

Dietary fiber   5.1   g 10%

Sugars   6.2   g 6.9%

Cholesterol   0.0   mg 0.0%

127.   Salmon-spinach rolls

Side dish, Fish, Low carbohydrate, Sugar free

Preparation time: 160 minutes

Number of people: 12

Ingredients

2 medium eggs

250 g frozen spinach, thawed

200 g grated cheese, 30+

200 g dairy spread with herbs, light

100 g salmon, smoked

Pepper

Preparation

Mix 2 eggs with 250 g of thawed frozen spinach and season with pepper.

Spread the mixture on a baking sheet covered with baking paper.

Sprinkle with 200 g of grated 30+ cheeses and bake for approx. 20 minutes in a preheated oven at 180 ° C.

Allow the mixture to cool and brush with 200 g light dairy spread with herbs.

Cover with 100 g of smoked salmon.

Roll it up carefully, wrap in aluminum foil and place in the fridge for about 2 hours.

Cut the roll into 12 pieces.

Nutritional values per person

Carbohydrates 1.2 g of

which sugars 1 g

Fat 7.7 g of

which saturated 4.1 g

Protein 10 g

Fiber 0.6 g

Vegetables 20 g

Kcal 115

Salt 0.78 g

Extract and Basic Nutrition Principles

Keto program, slimming this diet, low carb. When over such a diet, the body will regain its internal reserves, which will begin to use oil for energy.

The main emphasis is made on nutritional products with high-fat content. As you know, a balanced diet should consume protein, fats and carbohydrates evenly, but if you lose excess weight, nutrition is necessary to get rid of the excess of internal. In this case, the keto diet implies a reduction in protein, almost complete lack of carbohydrates and concentration on fat. Achieve this selection of unique products.

Is there a diet that keto the extra weight the body loses at all costs? Due to the extraordinary power, it re-breaks down fat instead of carbohydrates as the main energy supplier used in oil and ketosis.

Run ketosis is possible except in the diet carbohydrates. When we eat, mainly carbohydrates, they produce glucose in our bodies; the body gets at all costs and energy for the desired life. Do you eliminate carbohydrates? The body finds a way to spend other backs.

When the lack of liver, ketones turn into fat, no carbohydrates, fat-like glucose, and they give you the necessary energy. The use of fat as the main energy supplier allows the body to lower the level of insulin and burn fat as quickly as possible.

Go status ketosis a few weeks. Not instantly. Through his insight, characteristic symptoms:

- you will not want to have;
- visible acetone smell, urine, sweat, and halitosis;
- a desire to urinate more often;
- In the mouth will be dry.

Ketosis status and the main rules to be followed in order to reach:

- Oils become the main energy source;
- Carbohydrate diet should be more than 100 g / day;
- Protein diet should be in 1.5 - 2 g, 1 kg body weight;
- Obligatory water regimen, - 2 to 4 days 1;
- Any snack;
- A small exercise, for example, jogging or walking in the evening;
- Keto diet for the use of strict products.

4 Stages

As said, splitting is not the primary source of energy like fat immediately. To do this, in the stage of time and transition period, places 4 of the body.

1. It's still glucose. Then passed the keto diet, sometimes half a day or a day until the body continues to consume glucose, roughly, inertia.

2.   48 hours glycogen. After the body uses glucose, it undertakes to spend glycogen reserves, thcir muscles, and liver. It's two days.

3.   Recycle protein and fat. The most challenging stage in the transition process used fatty acid and energy for muscle fibers.

4.   Consumption of fat. Finally, the fourth stage - ketosis. The body gets used only to consume minimal amounts of fat carbohydrates, and burning protein in this context slows down and accelerates the use of fatty acids on the contrary.

The percentage seems to be the ketogenic diet on PFC:

· Oil - 60 - 75%;
· Protein - 25 - 35%;
· Carbohydrates - 10%.

Keto Diets Of Different Kinds

There are three types of keto diets, and each one uses the approach to nutrition.

- Classic keto diet. It is standard or permanent. Carbohydrate diet is not for everyone, a great time to minimize and only physically active people with permanent loads, for example, athletes. The diet adapts to low carbohydrate amount and average exercise intensity individually and only under expert care.
- Power keto diet. He is not targeted or targeted. This type of carbohydrate is used before an exercise, but their number should be significantly less than you could spend on exercise. Such a diet is easier to deal with, requiring great physical strength, especially those who have previously had plenty of carbohydrates.

· Cyclic keto diet. The meaning of this approach is a change in the power of carbohydrates and without them. A person is selected frequency and duration of carbohydrate supply. For example, 2 weeks of diet fat and protein, and the next 2 weeks carbohydrates. This allows you to replenish glycogen and take important trace elements. An excellent option for the most intense workouts. Again, under expert care.

Benefits

Why so many fans of keto nutrition? Also, they like, among experts, as well as western stars.

· Lose weight. Yes, such a diet, overall comprehensive full serving, lose fat. It is considered and nutritionists and experienced athletes. It can remove a short time, much fat. This loss of muscle mass can often be seen in hungry diets.

Keto practically, even for those who are unsuitable regularly, but after the diet must work especially carefully.

- Always fed. Food, which feed keto diet, is high calorie because hunger is not felt. Needless to say, this method is less painful, and food is drawn to plan like this.

- You can stimulate diabetes. As stated, when passing fats in the body is reduced sugar. You know for certain that high blood sugar triggers, diabetes is a second stage, especially genetic predisposition. In this case, a cleverly built diet will help to prevent the miscarriage of this disease.

- If you are improving pressure and casting to healthy cholesterol. Those who adhere to the keto-power, celebrate, blood pressure returns to normal. It becomes involved and slimming itself, cleaning up the risk of hypertension.

- You brain for improvement. It turns out that ketones, as a source of energy, can increase concentration and increase everyday intellectual activity. So, a diet is not only useful athletes but also intellectually active.
- Your skin will recover. She seems to be shining and looks younger. An overall improvement of the skin condition occurs in the background to reduce milk and dairy products and carbohydrates. According to some sources, it is responsible for the two product categories, bad skin.

Given that all positive diets recognize a significant portion of keto, nutritionists took another reason to treat pediatric epilepsy. Doctors say that in children with diet is reduced; the frequency of seizures, itself and the degree of the disease is reduced, to allow epileptic less medication.

Drawbacks

And yet, all the obvious benefits of the keto diet, there are some drawbacks. Mostly it is due to the symptoms of the synthesis of fatty acids. This phenomenon is known as keto-influenza. Side effects that may occur:

- Swelling;
- Constipation;
- Heartburn;
- Nausea;
- Headache;
- Fatigue;
- Heart palpitations;
- Seizures.

It must be said that you lose weight and quit smoking foods that are high in carbohydrates in any case of these symptoms even if you are on another diet.

The unpleasant side effects are the last 4 - 5 days, and you will never have a complete makeover. To avoid too bright signs to clear the products carbohydrate diet gradually, not suddenly.

Select Products For The Menu
Which products are suitable for the transition keto a diet?

Proteins: egg, steak, tuna, salmon, turkey, sardine, chicken, and so on.

The selection of vegetables is huge: ending from sprouts, all kinds of cabbage, cucumber, eggplant, and green leaf.

One is herbal, including all kinds of drinks, coffee teas, but no sweetener.

As spices are usually ginger, mustard, lemon, fresh and dried spices, without additives.

Weekly Menu
When designing the menu plan, remember that the products should contain the least carbohydrates, but not the most fat. Here are some ideas for each meal:

- Breakfast: scrambled eggs, onions, and cheese; a slice of salmon half avocado and poached egg; cheese pancakes without flour.

- Lunch: chicken salad; special keto salad; vegetable stew, soup, and dumplings; pate.
- Dinner: baked mushrooms; bacon, green beans for garnish; with a piece of pork, mozzarella.

About a week menu:

Monday:

- Fish souffle, toast, and a piece of cheese.
- Chicken breast, steamed, vegetable salad.
- Chicken meatballs, porridge.

Tuesday:

- One serving of cheese, baked apple.
- Chicken soup and broccoli, brown rice, water.
- Spinach salad, cheese, and assorted nuts.

Wednesday:

- Casserole with cheese and fresh berries.
- Rolls with ham and cheese and stewed vegetables.
- Boiled chicken pieces with zucchini.

Thursday:

- Omelet addition with cheese and bacon.
- Salmon, cooked, steamed, and stew vegetables.
- Fatty yogurt addition with nuts and fresh berries.

Friday:

- Portion of cottage cheese with sour cream.
- Soup-mashed cauliflower.
- Salmon fish in foil and boiled brown rice.

Saturday:

- Lemon cake.

- Vegetable soup and chicken dumplings with toast, butter, and cheese.
- Avocado and lettuce.

Market:

- Chicken breast, boiled egg.
- Veal pate, vegetable soup.
- Pork cutlet with mushroom sauce and asparagus.

Recipes

The menu offered includes a lot of simple dishes in the composition, but that does not mean that you should eat sparse and without diversity. Below recipes are the most popular food keto diets.

Special Bread

The recipe of this bread is perfect for keto power. This improved both the first and second dishes.

Requirements:

- ¼ Tablespoons. almond flour;
- 3 raw egg whites;
- 2 tsp. baking powder;
- 1 tsp. sea salt;
- 2 teaspoons apple cider vinegar;
- ¼ Tablespoons. water;
- 2 tablespoons sesame seeds.

Eat:

Until the oven is overheated to 175 degrees, stir the entire dry compound in the bowl, adding them protein and vinegar. Everything mix mixer. Preheat the water, top up the weight and mix until the dough is quite solid for modeling. Soak your hands with water and sow the dough cooling. The easiest way to use it for roasting. Put bread on the pan. Note that butter is greased on the baking sheet. Sprinkle bread, sesame seeds and bake for 1 hour

Stew Chicken with Olives And Cheese

Returns very tasty chicken, especially if you like black olives and feta cheese. And again in this recipe used sauce Pesto.

Requirements:

- 700 g of chicken meat;
- 1,5 tablespoons. whipped cream;
- 8 tablespoons of olives;
- 250 g cheese, white cheese;
- 100 g of sauce «Pesto»;
- 60 g vegetable oil;
- a clove of garlic;
- Spices and herbs taste.

Eat:

Boil chicken. Get a better chicken breast. Chop appropriate parts in case of preparation. Chop the garlic. Mix the sauce and cream. Lubricate the chicken into the oven dish, and then put the chicken pieces over it and then the olive. Sprinkle spices and pour garlic and creamy sauce. Bake inside the oven at 200 degrees for 30 minutes.

Salad with Avocado, Cheese, and Spinach

Thanks to the most delicious ingredients based on a hearty salad diet you will feel even.

Requirements:

70 grams of cheese;

50 g avocado;

150 g spinach;

a handful of nuts;

50 g bacon;

Olive oil.

Eat:

Chop the bacon into plates and fry in butter until a golden crust appears. Finely chop the spinach and grate the cheese. Stir in bacon, cheese, and spinach, add the composition of crushed nuts and stir in a spoon of olive oil.

Broccoli and Cheese

For those who are gentle and also rich in food, these two ingredients - hard cheese and broccoli.

Requirements:

- 400 g broccoli;
- 200 g cheese;
- 4 eggs;
- 100 onions;
- 40 g of butter.

Eat:

Chop blossom into broccoli and boiled, slightly salty. After 15 minutes, drain the boiling water and allow cooling. Chop the onions in half rings and fry the golden crust until displayed in butter in a pan for 5 minutes. At this stage, add the broccoli into pieces and fry for a few more minutes. Break the eggs directly in a pan and stir onions and broccoli gently. Simmer for 15 minutes over medium heat. Add the plate and cheese to the decision of preparation, it melted.

Omelets, No Food Intake

Traditionally, scrambled eggs, food, breakfast, but why to do it, for lunch or dinner? The mushrooms and bacon you get with are particularly delicious.

Requirements:

- 4 eggs;
- 30 g of dried mushrooms;
- 120 g bacon;
- 60 g hard cheese;
- Olive oil.

Eat:

Mushrooms pre-soak, warm water, and slice them soft and preparation julienne. Beat the eggs separately, and send them, warmed them, in a pan with olive oil. In the process add mushrooms, diced bacon and any spices, when the omelet was no longer ready, just grilled cheese on the pan. Let him wait a minute, and you can eat.

What is effective in losing weight

Studying the data of the studies, one can notice reliable facts that indicate stable and effective results of the ketogenic diet in the field of weight loss. People who tried to lose weight with her help were able to lose much more pounds than those who chose low-fat methods of losing weight.

The main reasons for the effectiveness of this system should include:

- The use of proteins, which act as the main helpers of a person in the process of losing weight.
- Gluconeogenesis is a condition where proteins and fats gradually become carbohydrates, which allows you to burn extra calories.
- Significant decrease in appetite. This is done by normalizing the level of hormones such as leptin and ghrelin.

- The emergence of insulin sensitivity. This phenomenon increases the metabolic rate, contributing to the maximum breakdown of fat.

Benefits for Diabetics

People who know firsthand about the metabolic syndrome try to grab onto any diet that can at least help a little. The popular keto-nutrition helps to cope with this metabolic syndrome, leading to metabolic disorders, the appearance of obesity, heart failure, and diabetes.

The main signs of metabolic syndrome include:

- A sharp increase in pressure;
- increased blood glucose;
- non-compliance with lipid indicators.

By timely abandoning bad habits and reviewing your diet, you will be able to get rid of the above symptoms. A ketogenic diet also plays an important role here. Experts have proven that it can increase insulin sensitivity by almost 70%. Some diabetics have even been able to refuse medication. The lipid profile improved, the level of triglycerides decreased to 80 mg/dl. The human body is gradually saturated with healthy fats.

As a result of this, the body manages to receive additional support from ketone bodies, which have useful properties.

Contraindications and complications

A ketogenic diet is not recommended if there are the following diseases:

Severe diabetes mellitus;

- kidney disease, liver;
- progressive encephalopathy;
- diseases of the heart and vascular system;
- cerebrovascular disease.

Adverse reactions to this diet can be:

- Hair loss. This is quite possible as a result of a deficiency of mineral elements in the selected diet.
- Growth lag.
- An increase in cholesterol. If such a picture is observed, then it is necessary to reduce the proportion of fats to other substances, for example, 70/30. This will provide acceptable cholesterol values.
- Renal calculi as a result of drinking large volumes of fluid. To avoid this, it is important to periodically pass urine for analysis and an ultrasound of the kidneys.
- Drowsiness, lethargic state.
- Constipation If there are prerequisites for their occurrence, it is better to increase the amount of fluid drunk.
- Excess weight. This condition is rare, but the menu still requires adjustment.
- A sharp loss of kilograms. If weight loss is carried out to normal aisles, then this is completely considered

the norm. But there are times when a person continues to lose weight to critical boundaries; then, it is necessary to radically change the constituent elements of his nutrition, choosing the ideal option.

How to minimize risks

The ketone diet is safe for humans. But still, there are cases of side effects during the period of adaptation of the body.

To avoid this from occurring, you can do a little training by trying a low-carb diet first. Its main goal is the minimum intake of carbohydrates for two weeks.

Also, as a result of the introduction of a ketogenic diet, the mineral balance in the body can change. That is why it is crucial to add the necessary minerals (sodium, potassium, magnesium) to the menu.

Sometimes during the diet, an undesirable and clearly noticeable smell of acetone from the mouth appears. It will be possible to correct the situation by increasing the volume of drinking water or using chewing gums.

More Health Benefits Of The Keto Diet

The Keto diet was initially been a method to treat neurological diseases, such as epilepsy.

Studies have shown that the diet can provide benefits for a wide range of different health problems:

- Heart problems: The ketogenic diet can include risk factors such as for overweight, HDL cholesterol values, blood pressure, including blood sugar.
- Cancer: The diet is used to treat different types and to reduce the growth of a tumor.
- Alzheimer's: The ketogenic diet can potentially reduce Alzheimer's symptoms and reduce progression.
- Epilepsy: Researcher has shown that the ketogenic diet can lead to a significant reduction in seizures in children.

- Parkinson's: A study found that it improves the symptoms of Parkinson's
- Polycystic ovarian syndrome: The ketogenic diet can help reduce insulin levels, which may play a significant role in polycystic ovarian syndrome.
- Brain damage: an animal study has found that the ketogenic diet can help to reduce concussion and help to repair brain damage.
- Acne: Lower insulin levels and less sugar and processed food can greatly reduce acne.

However, it must be borne within mind that studies in all these areas are far from conclusive.

A ketogenic diet can provide many health benefits, especially in metabolic, neurological, and insulin-related diseases.

Food To Avoid On The Keto Diet

You should shun foods that are high in carbohydrates.

Below is a list of foods that should be reduced or eliminated on a ketogenic diet:

- Sugar-rich food: Soft drinks, fruit drinks, smoothies, candy, ice cream, etc.
- Cereals and starches: Food based on wheat, rice, pasta, bread, breakfast cereals, etc.
- Fruit : All types of fruit, except small portions of berries or strawberries.
- Beans and carbohydrate-rich vegetables: Peas, brown beans, lentils, chickpeas, and so on.
- Root vegetables and the tubers: Potatoes, carrots, parsnip, etc.
- Low fat and diet products: These are often processed and high in carbohydrates.
- Certain herbs and sauces: These often contain sugar and unhealthy fats.

- Unhealthy fats: Processed and heated vegetable oils.
- Alcohol: Many alcoholic beverages will get you from ketosis due to the high carbohydrate content.
- Sugar-free diet products: These are often high in sugar alcohols, which may affect your ketone level. In addition, these products are often processed.
- Avoid carbohydrate-rich foods such as grains, sugar, fruit, vegetables, juices, and fruit.

Food To Eat On The Keto Diet

The Keto diet will largely consist of food on the list below:

- Meat: Steak, ham, bacon, sausage, chicken, and lime cake.
- Fatty fish: Salmon, herring, mackerel, eel.
- Eggs: Free-range eggs rich in omega-3.

- Butter and cream: Grass-fed when possible.
- Cheese: Unprocessed, preferably from grass-fed cows.
- Nuts and seeds: Almonds, walnuts, linseed, pumpkin seeds, chia seeds, etc.
- Healthy oils: Extra virgin olive oil, avocado oil, coconut oil.
- Avocados: Fresh. preferably organic avocados.
- Carbohydrate poor vegetables: Most green vegetables, tomatoes, onion in moderation, peppers.
- Spices: Salt, pepper, low carbohydrate spices

It is good to opt for a diet based on whole foods with one ingredient.

Base the vast majority of your diet on foods such as fish, egg, meat, butter, nuts, healthy oils, avocados, and many low-carbohydrate vegetables.

Healthy Keto Snacks

Supposing you get hungry in between meals, you can always have a healthy Keto snack in between:

- Fat meat or fish
- Cheese
- Hand nuts
- Cheese with olives
- Cooked eggs
- 90% dark chocolate
- Low-carbohydrate milkshake with almond milk, cocoa, and nut butter
- Cottage cheese with peanut butter and cocoa powder.
- Strawberries with cream
- Celery with salsa and guacamole
- Small portions of meals
- Good snacks for a keto diet include pieces of cheese, olives, meat, eggs, nuts, and dark chocolate.

How You Can Eat On A Keto Diet

It is not very difficult to eat ketogenic when you eat out.

Most restaurants do have meat or fish on the menu. You can order this and have the carbohydrate food replaced by extra vegetables and meat.

Egg-based meals are also a good option, such as an omelet or eggs with bacon or sausages.

Another favorite is hamburgers without a sandwich. Have the fries replaced with vegetables. Have extra avocado, cheese, bacon, or eggs serve. Also, be careful with sauces; these often contain sugar.

At the restaurant, you can always ask for extra meat, cheese, guacamole, or cream.

For dessert, you can choose cheeses, olives or berries with cream

When you are out for dinner, choose a dish based on meat, fish, or eggs. Request extra vegetables instead of bread, fries, or other carbohydrate-rich foods to make cheese or cream as a dessert.

Side Effects Of The Keto Diet And How To Limit Them

Although the keto diet is safe for healthy people, side effects (especially in the beginning) can occur while your body adjusts.

This is mainly known as the keto flu and usually passes after a few days.

During the keto flu, you often have little energy, and you function less mentally. You may be more hungry (especially for carbohydrates), sleep problems, nausea, bowel problems, and reduced sports performance.

To minimize this, you can start with a healthy diet with reduced carbohydrates. This way, your body can get used to burning more fat before you scrape off almost all carbs.

A ketogenic diet can change the water and mineral balance in your body. Adding extra salt and minerals to your diet can help you.

Add minerals to your diet, 3,000 to 4,000 mg of sodium, 1,000 mg of potassium, including 300 mg of magnesium each day to minimize side effects.

Especially in the beginning, it is important that you eat until you are no longer hungry and do not pay much attention to a calorie restriction. In most cases, weight loss also happens without paying attention to your calories.

Most side effects of a ketogenic diet can be limited. Gradual starting and mineral supplements can support you in this.

Nutritional Supplements On A Keto Diet
Nutritional supplements are not necessary on the Keto diet but can support them.

MCT oil: MCT oil contains energy and helps to increase the number of ketones. You can add this to drinks, cottage cheese, and yogurt.

Minerals: Add sodium, magnesium to maintain your body's mineral balance.

Caffeine: Caffeine has positive properties in terms of energy, fat loss, and performance.

Exogenous ketones: This supplement can help you produce more ketones.

Creatine: Creatine can help you improve your performance.

Whey: Supports your protein intake.

Certain supplements can be very beneficial on a ketogenic diet. Think of MCT oil, exogenous ketones, and minerals.

Frequently Asked Questionsconcerning a ketogenic diet

1. Can I ever eat carbohydrates again?

Yes. However, it is important to limit your carbohydrate intake very much in the beginning. After the first 2-3 months, you can occasionally eat carbohydrates. It is important that you immediately pick up the diet again.

2. Will I lose muscle mass?

There is a possiblilty that you will lose muscle mass on every diet. However, the high amount of protein in combination with many ketones in the body will minimize the loss of muscle mass, particularly if you do strength training.

3. Can I build muscle mass on a ketogenic diet?

Yes, but this may not work as well as on a moderate carbohydrate diet.

4. Do I have to eat carbs every now and then?

No. However, a few days high in calories are beneficial every now and then.

5. How many proteins can you eat?

Protein consumption must be moderate. Too high a protein intake can cause your insulin to the peak. About 35% of the total calories is the maximum.

6. What should I do if I am constantly tired, weak, or exhausted?

You are probably not yet completely in ketosis, or you are not yet effectively burning fat. To counter this, you can reduce carbohydrates and go over the points above. A supplement such as MCT oil or exogenous ketones can help.

7. My urine smells strange. Why is this so?

No alarm. This is due to the separation of substances that are produced during ketosis.

8. My breath stinks. What can I do about this?

This is a common side effect. Drink more water, take sugar-free chewing gum, or brush your teeth.

9. Being in ketosis would be dangerous. Is this true?

People often confuse ketosis with ketoacidosis. The first is, of course, the second occurs with uncontrolled diabetes.

Ketoacidosis is dangerous, while ketosis is normal and healthy during a ketogenic diet.

10. I have bowel problems and diarrhea. What can I do?

This is a common complaint that usually passes after 3 to 4 weeks. If it continues, you can add a little more fiber-rich vegetables to your diet. Magnesium supplements can help with constipation.

A Keto Diet Does Miracles, But Not For Everyone

The Keto diet can do much good for overweight people, diabetics, or people who want to improve their metabolic health.

It may be less suitable for top athletes or people who want to gain large amounts of muscle masses.

And, as with any diet, it only works with consistency and in the long run.

That said, few other methods with nutrition have as many health and weight loss benefits as the ketogenic diet.

Good Things To Save At The Supermarket

If you are thinking of buying some foods, opt for a small basket. A big cart will make you fill it. Choose it according to your needs!

Circulate clockwise

Did you know that the location of a grocery store entrance can have a significant effect on the way you shop? Access on the right will make you circulate counterclockwise. Studies show that consumers who travel in this direction spend, on average, $2 more than consumers who travel clockwise. Conversely, a door on the left will move you in the right direction, and you will save!

This is because customers who go to the left tend to focus more forward and less backward. They spend less time there, so fewer expenses. By placing the door on the right, grocery stores have noticed that they are doing better deals than those having access to the center or left.

The next time you go to the grocery store, turn left immediately to save a few dollars! Of course, not all grocery stores are built that way.

Do your shopping in U

Start your market in the fresh produce section and do the U: all the essential commodities are there, such as fruits and vegetables, dairy products, etc. If you start with the purchase of basic items, you will not have much room for unnecessary food in the center aisles.

Moreover, the most common way to get around the supermarket is to do the perimeter while browsing the different shelves, as needed.

Stick to the main aisles

In Canada, 71% of consumers walk all the aisles to make sure they do not forget anything. However, this is a waste of time and an obstacle to your savings. By performing each of the aisles, you will succumb to the temptation of commodities you do not need. Make a habit of visiting only the main ones, especially those on the outskirts.

Consider ugly foods

You will see more and more in Canadian supermarkets of deformed fruits and vegetables that are often ignored by consumers. Know that these small fruits and imperfect vegetables are sold 30% cheaper than those who are more beautiful.

For the moment, not all grocery stores offer them, but if you have the chance, try them! After all, it's not the appearance that counts, but the taste.

Know the meat and limit your consumption

Purchase less expensive cuts of meat such as lean ground meat, whole chicken, pork shank, and less tender cuts of meat.

Another solution is to reduce your consumption of red meat to lighten your bill. Lentils, tofu, quinoa, and beans are vegetable proteins that cost less and are worth discovering.

Check the expiry dates

First of all, it must be recognized that an expiry date does not necessarily mean that the food must be discarded as soon as it is "overdue." Often, these dates are only indicators to remind you when the product can be consumed at its fullest. That is, when the food is to its fullest taste, full texture, or nutritional value. However, care must be taken since the expiry date only applies when the product is not open. From the opening, the date no longer applies.

At the grocery store, there is nothing stopping you from picking up the items from the bottom to get food, the date of which is as far away as possible. They will be better longer, and you will avoid food waste.

Look at the bottom and top shelves

When next you visit the grocery store, notice that the most popular and expensive products are placed at the height of your eyes. Make a habit of looking at the top shelves, where the lesser-known are and often more affordable commodities and lower shelves, which usually have staple foods.

Fewer than one in two checks the quantity information when making purchases. However, the first thing to do is to compare the price of items of the same nature. Taking two blocks of cheese and choosing the cheapest is not necessarily the best deal. It is necessary to know how to compare the price to the unit of measure, either by 100 g or 100 ml and not only the selling price. To quickly compare different formats, consult the tablet label, the price per unit of measure is still listed.

Increasingly, consumers are confused at the variety of formats present. They have trouble figuring out which product is the cheapest. Often, this will lead them to choose products on sale. However, these are not necessarily cheaper than those posted at current prices. Even for products you regularly buy, always evaluate the unit price. That's the thing.

Beware of large formats

What about family, jumbos, and economic formats? At first glance, they seem more profitable. However, it is not always true to think that large formats are more interesting than small ones. To be certain, follow the trick: consult the label of the price per unit, either by 100 g or 100 ml and compare!

Also, be aware that just getting bigger sizes can push you to increase portions. As a result, your family box could very well empty as quickly as if you had bought the small format. Result: the economy is no longer there!

Minimize individual packages

As they are very practical, we often tend to minimize the amount of individual packaging we buy. Whether it's a small container of yogurt, compote, juice, or a packaged cake, these products generally have a much higher unit price. Of course, these products represent a winning solution for families. With lunches and children, single servings remain very convenient, and we are ready to pay a little more.

On the other hand, if time permits, the solution is to turn to bulk foods or bigger sizes (if, of course, it's better) and makes small individual portions in advance. In this way, you can dose portions yourself, and it will be more convenient when you make the lunches. Consider this tip for your next meal planning!

Alter the different brands in your basket

In the past, private labels were often viewed negatively by consumers. Rumor had it that the products we're selling at a lower price because of poorer quality compared to the private label. Now, people are finding that food is just as delicious and, above all, more affordable. Home brands are much improved and have increased their quality standard.

Adopt frozen fruits and vegetables

A frozen food section is an interesting option for your budget. This section allows you to enjoy good fruits and vegetables throughout the year, and at a reasonable price. However, choose blends in their natural state, without adding salt, fat, or sugar.

Claim a deferred coupon

A product is announced in a circular, and it remains in the display? Do not be shy and ask for your postponement: you are entitled to it. Also, know that it is valid at all times.

In addition, if the item is no longer available, supermarkets must offer something of the same nature and the same price.

Take a look at the time of the transaction

The last step before you proclaim pro supermarket is always to check the registration of your products at the checkout. Would you not want to break all your efforts into a simple price error? Too often, it is these small blunders that ruin your savings. Please note that according to the price accuracy policy, when there is an error, and the item is less than $ 10, the merchant must give you the product free of charge.

In the end, double-check your grocery bill.

Small impulsive fishing: stay tuned!

Good smells

The moment you walk at the front door of your supermarket, a good smell of roast chicken tickles your nostrils. Do you know that this smell could make you spend more? According to a study carried out, adding odors in a store increases purchase intentions by 80%.

Why do you feel a good fresh bread automatically make you want to buy some? Odors are directly related to the part of the brain where the emotions sit. In addition, the brain analyzes perfumes without our being aware of them, and this significantly influences our purchasing behavior.

Of course, few people do not like to smell freshly baked bread. It's more pleasant to do your market when it smells good. Just be aware of the smells that sometimes lead to unplanned purchases.

The music

At the grocery store, a customer stops about three seconds in an alley to make his choice. Do you know that this figure can vary according to the musical rhythm broadcast in supermarkets? Indeed, the more the melody is slow and pleasant, the more you will move slowly and, at the same time, the more you will spend. For example, you will think more about the choices to make; you will analyze the promotional posters, you will take the time to read the labels, etc.

On the other hand, if your grocery store plays fast music, you will be inclined to impulsive purchases. In either case, try to keep the focus on your grocery list. If you wish, bring your own music!

The stickers

The allegations as 100% natural, made with real fruit, light, with added calcium, fat, etc. are all indicators that reassure us as a consumer. However, focusing on one of these criteria is distracting from nutrition information.

A box of cookies that displays without trans-fat, cholesterol, and low saturated fat is still a fat and sweet product. However, the health criteria mentioned in large print make us forget the other nutritional characteristics of the product. This is confusing to the consumer who always wants to make the best choices.

The solution is to take the time to read the labels and the list of ingredients. Try not to buy products whose list contains words that are too complicated to pronounce. The important thing is to choose foods that have the fewest ingredients possible.

In addition, compare the products with each other: the original product and the one with 40% less fat, for example. A "light" food does not mean it is healthier because to make it less fat, some manufacturers often compensate with sugar or other harmful ingredients to maintain texture and taste.

The discounts 2 for 1, 3 for 5

Supermarkets sometimes offer types of discounts that encourage consumers to buy beyond their needs. Balances such as three canned soups for $5 are a good example, as they can make you want to automatically take three when in reality, you only need two. Remember that in most grocery stores, prices are set individually. If you buy only one item, you will only pay for that quantity.

Tasting kiosks

Who has never been tempted by a bite to eat at the tasting booth? These small stands are a real cute catch! Of course, you do not have to do without it ... It's still a little grocery. On the other hand, we must know that this sometimes pushes us to make unexpected purchases. Stay alert and ask yourself the question: do I really need this week?

Tastings are a good way to discover new products and vary the menus. If you like the product you like, it will still be possible to get it the following week. As a bonus, they sometimes offer discounts or coupons to use at the next purchase. This is a double reason to wait until later to switch to a planned purchase mode!

Displays

Grocery stores like to create displays of products by association, that is to say, by making special arrangements such as a "special Italy" with pasta and sauces, chocolate for fondue near berries or salad vinaigrette near the vegetables. On the one hand, it enhances food while suggesting combinations of ideas to consumers. On the other hand, it may encourage us to go beyond our needs. Often, these products are not necessarily on sale. We must remain vigilant!

Conclusion

The keto diet is a high protein diet, which can be very suitable for the elderly because it helps us avoid losing muscle mass. In addition to proteins of animal origin, such as red meat or chicken, eggs or fish, it gives preference to proteins of plant origin such as legumes or nuts.

Despite its indisputable nutritional value, the keto diet avoids fruits, due to its high sugar content, and gives preference to vegetables as a source of fibre, especially those that grow above the ground, which usually has lower carbohydrate content carbon than those that grow under it, such as potatoes, onions or carrots. Although the keto diet will help you lose weight quickly, the studies are inconclusive about maintaining that weight loss.

The ketogenic diet can help us to alleviate or even avoid many ailments that can occur in old age. It is important, especially in old age, to take care of the appropriate supplementation during a ketogenic diet, so that, for example, the muscles do not lose more than they normally do and to relieve symptoms such as keto flu. The earlier you start a healthy diet, the better for quality of life in old age. And when we write about healthy eating, of course we immediately think of the ketogenic diet!

CPSIA information can be obtained
at www.ICGtesting.com
Printed in the USA
LVHW081331260121
677539LV00005B/23

9 781801 271158